FUNDAMEN
OF RAD

CH00685415

IS Francis, FRCS, MBBS, BDS (Hons)
*Department of Radiology, The Royal Free Hospital,
Hampstead, London, UK*

RI Aviv, MRCP, MBChB
*Department of Radiology, The Royal Free Hospital,
Hampstead, London, UK*

EA Dick, MRCP, MBBS, BSc (Hons)
*Department of Radiology, The Royal Free Hospital,
Hampstead, London, UK*

Editor
AF Watkinson, FRCS, FRCR
*Department of Radiology, The Royal Free Hospital,
Hampstead, London, UK*

R E M E D I C A
P U B L I S H I N G

Printed in Great Britain by The Bath Press
Published by
REMEDICA Publishing Limited
32-38 Osnaburgh Street
London, NW1 3ND, UK
Tel: +44 171 388 7677
Fax: +44 171 388 7678
E-mail: info@remedica.com

ISBN 1 901346 01 3

Preface

Fundamental Aspects of Radiology

This book evolved out of our need to assimilate information that we had not previously encountered in our medical training. It aims to cover all aspects of physics, anatomy and pharmacology as related to radiology. In covering these areas, it should serve as a useful basis for revision for the Part I Fellowship examination in Radiology. In addition, it should prove useful as a basic text for all radiologists and radiographers in training, both within and outside the United Kingdom.

The ever-expanding role of imaging within medicine means that radiology is playing an increasing part in both undergraduate and postgraduate medical examinations. This book provides an up-to-date overview of radiological physics and anatomy that should be of use to medical students, as well as to the interested clinician.

IS Francis
RI Aviv
EA Dick

July 1999

Acknowledgements

We wish to thank the radiologists and radiographers at the Royal Free Hospital who have helped us in obtaining and producing the many images contained within this book.

Particular thanks should be given to Dr Robert Speller, who kindly and constructively reviewed much of the physics sections. We are grateful to Liz Roberts for her invaluable secretarial skills, as well as to all at REMEDICA for their support and enthusiasm throughout this project.

Foreword

Fundamental Aspects of Radiology

When radiologists-in-training first enter the speciality they are usually overwhelmed by the largely unfamiliar environment and, for them, the variety of new knowledge expected. They have to learn large amounts of factual information, acquire technical skills, and learn to integrate clinical data with the appearances on imaging examinations. A knowledge of normal anatomy, basic physics, radiation protection and equipment design is essential. These topics are, of course, the subjects of written examinations. This book, written by recent examination candidates and edited by an experienced radiologist, will help future candidates prepare for the first part of the examination for the Fellowship of the Royal College of Radiologists and similar examinations in other countries. It provides the equivalent of detailed lecture notes and, in providing an overview of the various subjects, a framework for in-depth study of individual topics. I hope the book proves useful to all concerned and wish it every success.

Peter Armstrong
Professor of Radiology
St. Bartholomew's Hospital, London, UK

To our families

Contents

Section One: **Anatomy**

Section Two: **Basic Physics**

Section Three: Modality-Based Physics

Section Four: Pharmacology of Radiology

Fundamental Aspects of Radiology

Section One

Anatomy

1.1 The Developing Foetus and Infant

Antenatal ultrasound

Foetal heart is first detected at 6-7 weeks (transvaginally at 5 weeks)

Age predictor	Useful range (weeks)	Accuracy (weeks)
Crown rump length	6-12	+/- 1
Biparietal diameter	12-30	+/- 2
Femur length	14-22	+/- 2
Abdominal circumference	30-40	+/- 4

Table 1.11 Time-frame of developmental observations

Gestational sac appears between 4 and 7 weeks
Yolk sac appears from 5 weeks onwards and disappears by week 11
Foetal pole is identified from 6 weeks onwards

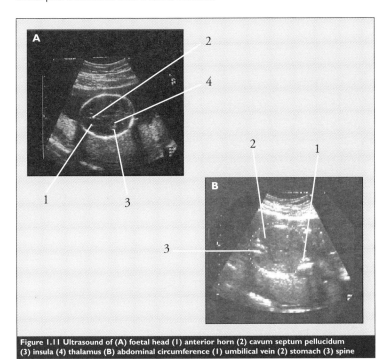

Figure 1.11 Ultrasound of (A) foetal head (1) anterior horn (2) cavum septum pellucidum (3) insula (4) thalamus (B) abdominal circumference (1) umbilical vein (2) stomach (3) spine

Foetal anatomy

Head/central nervous system (CNS)

Ventricular hemispheric ratio
Measure at the cavum septum pellucidum
Ratio should be <0.5
Foetal myelination begins at the brain stem and proceeds cranially
50% of newborn babies have a cavum septum pellucidum; 20% persist at 6 months

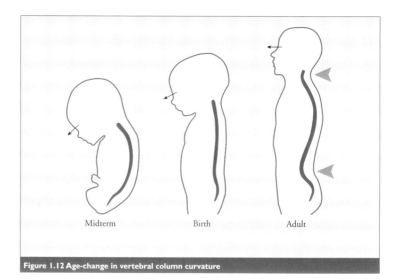

Midterm   Birth   Adult

Figure 1.12 Age-change in vertebral column curvature

In the foetus, there is only a primary curvature of the vertical column
Secondary curvature in the cervical and lumbar regions develops with function

Cardiovascular

Four chambers are visible at 14 weeks
Right ventricular wall thickness is greater than that of the left

Limbs

Visible at 7 weeks

Abdomen

Exomphalus from 6 to 11 weeks
Bowel returns with 270° anticlockwise rotation

Kidneys and adrenals

Visible from 14 and 20 weeks, respectively
Adrenals are initially one-third the size of the kidneys

Vascular tree
The two umbilical arteries become the medial umbilical ligaments
The median umbilical ligament is developed from the urachus

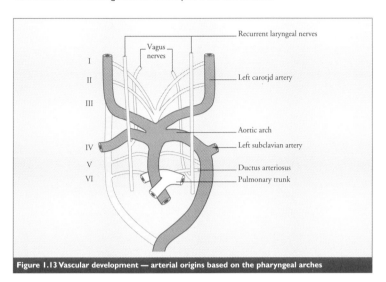

Figure 1.13 Vascular development — arterial origins based on the pharyngeal arches

The single umbilical vein becomes the ligamentum teres

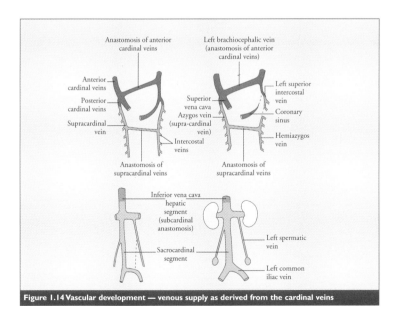

Figure 1.14 Vascular development — venous supply as derived from the cardinal veins

Bones
Bones that ossify in membrane are: skull vault, facial bones, clavicle
All other bones ossify in cartilage except the occipital and sphenoid
bones, which ossify in both membrane and cartilage

Skull (at birth)
Sutures are straight lines
Sinuses are not aerated
Wormian bones are present

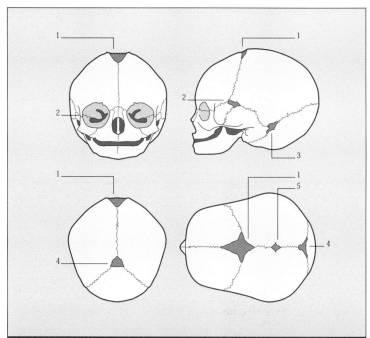

Figure 1.15 Anatomical drawings of infant skulls indicating fontanelles (1) anterior
(2) anterolateral (3) posterolateral (4) posterior (5) sagittal
Reprinted from Handbook of Neuroradiology: Brain & Skull (2nd Edition), Osborn & Tong, chapter 1, page 8: figure 1-3,
1996, by permission of Mosby.

Fontanelles
Anterior fontanelle closes at 2 years
Posterior fontanelle closes at 6 months
Lateral fontanelles close at 2-3 months

Greatest amount of skull growth is in the first year following birth
Complete growth occurs by 8 years of age

			Age of ossification (years, unless otherwise stated)
Arm			
Primary	Shaft of humerus, ulna and radius		8th week of foetal life
Secondary	Coracoid	Root	17
		Midportion	1
	Acromion		15-18
	Scapula and sternal end of clavicle		20
	Humerus	Greater tuberosity	3
		Lesser tuberosity	5
	Elbow	Capitellum	1
		Radius head	3
		Radius (distal)	1-2
		Internal (medial) epicondyle	5
		Trochlea	9-11
		Olecranon	9-11
		Ulna (distal)	5-8
		Lateral epicondyle	9-11
	Hand	Capitate and hamate	4 months
		Triquetral	3
		Lunate	4
		Trapezium/trapezoid/ scaphoid	6
		Pisiform	11
		Metacarpal heads before bases	2.5-3
		Bases of proximal phalanges before bases of mid and distal phalanges	2.5-3
Leg			
Primary	Bones of hip, femur and tibia		7th week of foetal life
	Fibula		8th week of foetal life
Secondary	Femur	Proximal	0.5-1
		Greater trochanter	3-5
		Lesser trochanter	8-14
		Distal	At birth
	Tibia	Proximal	At birth
		Tubercle	5-10
	Feet	Calcaneus and talus	6th month of foetal life
		Cuboid	At birth
		Navicular	3-4
		Cuneiform - medial	3
		- middle	3
		- lateral	1

Table 1.12 Ossification in the (A) arm and (B) leg of the developing foetus and infant

1.2 The Central Nervous System

Brain
Each cerebral hemisphere is divided into four lobes: frontal, parietal, temporal, occipital
Insula (of Reil) lies in the depth of the lateral ventricle
Operculum is the region of overlap of the parietal, frontal and temporal lobes

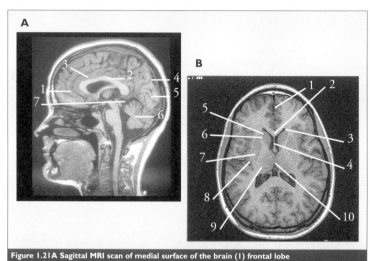

Figure 1.21A Sagittal MRI scan of medial surface of the brain (1) frontal lobe
(2) corpus callosum (3) cingulate gyrus (4) parieto-occipital fissure (5) occipital lobe
(6) cerebellum (7) quadrigeminal plate
Figure 1.21B Axial MRI through basal ganglia and internal capsule (1) interhemispheric fissure
(2) corpus callosum (3) anterior horn of lateral ventricle (4) septum pellucidum (5) head of
caudate nucleus (6) internal capsule (7) lentiform nucleus (8) external capsule (9) thalamus
(10) third ventricle

White-matter tracts
Commissural fibres
Link similar areas in the cerebral hemispheres
Examples: corpus callosum, anterior commissure, posterior commissure, habenular commissure

Arcuate fibres
Link gyri of one cerebral hemisphere
Examples: cingulum, fornix

Projection fibres
Connect the cortex to the lower parts of the brain and spinal cord
Examples: internal capsule, basal ganglia — caudate, amygdaloid, lentiform nucleus, claustrum

Ventricular system

Cerebrospinal fluid (CSF)-filled spaces

Two lateral ventricles expand into each cerebral hemisphere

The third ventricle, aqueduct and fourth ventricle are in the midline and in continuity with the third ventricle — normally these are all symmetrical and they are lined by ependyma and invaginated by blood vessels

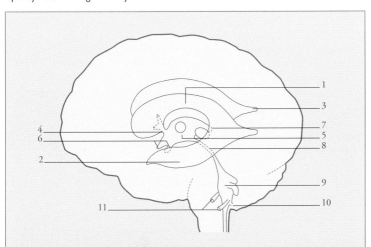

Figure 1.22 Anatomical drawing of the ventricular system (lateral view) (1) body, lateral ventricle (2) temporal horn, lateral ventricle (3) occipital horn, lateral ventricle (4) foramen of Monro (5) body, third ventricle (6) optic and infundibular recesses, third ventricle (7) suprapineal recess, third ventricle (8) aqueduct (9) body, fourth ventricle (10) foramen of Magendie (11) lateral recesses of fourth ventricle with foramina of Luschka
Reprinted from Handbook of Neuroradiology: Brain & Skull (2nd Edition), Osborn & Tong, chapter 2, page 20: figure 2-2, 1996, by permission of Mosby.

Ventricular size is assessed by:
 1. Evans ratio
 2. Maximum width of sellae median

CSF

150 ml produced daily by the choroid plexus (most is produced from within the lateral ventricle)

Flows cephalad from the basal cisterns

Flows caudally anterior to the spinal cord — cephalad posterior to the spinal cord

Relations of the ventricles

Lateral ventricle

Consists of a body, and temporal, frontal and occipital horns
The trigone represents the junction of the temporal and occipital horns

Superior	Corpus callosum
Inferior (medial to lateral)	Body of the caudate, thalamostriate groove, thalamus and fornix
Medial	Septum pellucidum
Lateral	Caudate nucleus

Table 1.21 Relations of the lateral ventricle

Third ventricle

Slit-like limited space

Superior (anterior to posterior)	Anterior comissure, fornix
Inferior	Supraoptic recess above chiasm, hypothalamus; infundibular recess superior to pituitary stalk
Anterior	Lamina terminalis (supraoptic recess above chiasm)
Posterior	Habenular and posterior commissure and pineal gland (suprapineal recess above this)
Lateral	Thalami

Table 1.22 Relations of the third ventricle

Fourth ventricle

Situated between the cerebellum and the posterior surface of the medulla oblongata and pons

Superior	Superior cerebellar peduncles; superior medullary velum
Floor	(Rhomboid fossa) Pons and medulla
Three apertures: Medial	Foramen of Magendie drains into the cisterna magna
Lateral	Two foramina of Luschka drain into the pontine cistern

Table 1.23 Relations of the fourth ventricle

Subarachnoid cisterns
CSF-filled spaces named according to the surrounding anatomical structures

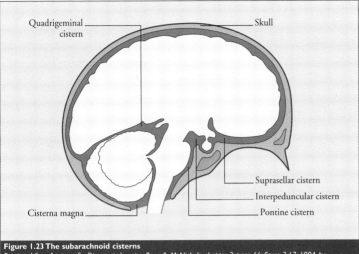

Figure 1.23 The subarachnoid cisterns
Reprinted from Anatomy for Diagnostic Imaging, Ryan & McNichols, chapter 2, page 66: figure 2.17, 1994, by permission of WB Saunders Company.

Pituitary gland
12 mm transverse diameter, 8 mm anteroposterior diameter
Anterior lobe is five times larger than the posterior lobe
Develops as an outpouching of Rathke's pouch
Blood supply is from the hypophyseal arteries (from the internal carotid artery)

Brain stem
Connects the cerebral hemispheres with the spinal cord
Consists of (superior to inferior) the midbrain, pons and medulla oblongata

Midbrain	Pons	Medulla oblongata
Related structures		
2 cerebral peduncles	Middle cerebellar peduncle	Pyramids
4 colliculae	Basilar artery	Olive
Superior cerebellar peduncles	Floor of IVth ventricle	Inferior cerebellar peduncle
		Floor of IVth ventricle
Cranial nerves		
II, III, IV	V, VI, VII, VIII	IX, X, XI, XII
CT level		
Circle of Willis	Anterior clivus	IVth ventricle
	Lateral petrous temporal bone	

Table 1.24 Characteristics of the midbrain, pons and medulla oblongata

Cerebellum

Contained within the posterior fossa below the tentorium cerebelli
Separated from the pons and midbrain by the fourth ventricle
Connected via three pairs of cerebellar peduncles
Vermix is the narrow midline portion

Blood supply

Posterior inferior cerebellar artery (PICA) — vertebral artery
Anterior inferior cerebellar artery (AICA) — basilar artery
Superior cerebellar artery — basilar artery

Normal intracranial calcification

Pineal gland

50% of adults have calcification
Marks the posterior margin of the third ventricle
Midline structure — a shift >3 mm is significant

Habenular commissure

Anterior to the pineal gland
Forms a reverse 'C'

Glomus of the choroid plexus (within the lateral ventricles)

Usually symmetrical and bilateral

Dura mater

Interclinoid and petroclinoid ligaments

Basal ganglia

Affects all subcortical gray matter except the red nucleus

Internal carotid artery (ICA)

Lens of the eye

Vascular supply to the brain
Arterial
Supplied by branches of the ICA and vertebrobasilar system

ICA
Very tortuous with six bends and can be subdivided into:
1. Intracranial portion
   ophthalmic artery
   thalamic artery
   posterior communicating artery
   anterior choroidal artery
   anterior cerebral artery (Heubener recurrent artery, anterior
   communicating artery, frontopolar, callosomarginal and pericallosal artery)
   middle cerebral artery (medial and lateral lenticulostriate, cortical
   branches)
2. Carotid syphon
   no branches
3. Cavernous portion
   meningohypophyseal artery
4. Petrous portion
   producing the pterygoid artery
5. Cervical portion

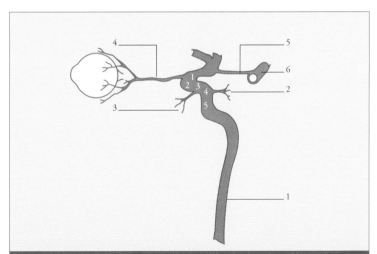

**Figure 1.24 Lateral view of the internal carotid artery ICA and its branches: white numbers
denote carotid segments (see text); blue numbers (1) cervical ICA (2) meningohypophyseal trunk
(3) lateral mainstem artery (4) ophthalmic artery (5) posterior communicating artery
(6) posterior cerebral artery**
*Reprinted from Handbook of Neuroradiology: Brain & Skull (2nd Edition), Osborn & Tong, chapter 4, page 40: figure
4-1, 1996, by permission of Mosby.*

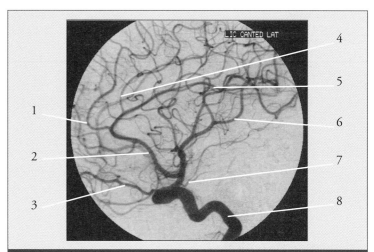

Figure 1.25 Lateral view of carotid angiogram (1) frontopolar artery (2) anterior cerebral artery (3) ophthalmic artery (4) callosomarginal artery (5) pericallosal artery (6) middle cerebral artery (7) anterior choroidal artery (8) internal carotid artery

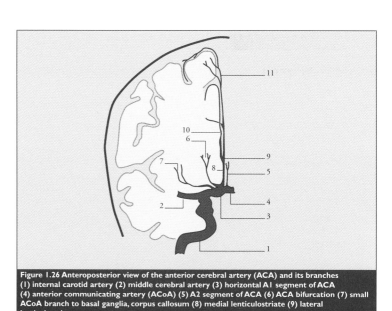

Figure 1.26 Anteroposterior view of the anterior cerebral artery (ACA) and its branches (1) internal carotid artery (2) middle cerebral artery (3) horizontal A1 segment of ACA (4) anterior communicating artery (ACoA) (5) A2 segment of ACA (6) ACA bifurcation (7) small ACoA branch to basal ganglia, corpus callosum (8) medial lenticulostriate (9) lateral lenticulostriate
(10) pericallosal artery (11) callosomarginal artery
Reprinted from Handbook of Neuroradiology: Brain & Skull (2nd Edition), Osborn & Tong, chapter 5, page 52: figure 5-2, 1996, by permission of Mosby.

Cavernous sinus
III, IV, V1 and V2 cranial nerves in lateral wall
VI cranial nerve lies inferior
Supraclinoid ICA lies medial to the clinoid process and inferolateral to the optic
nerve and canal

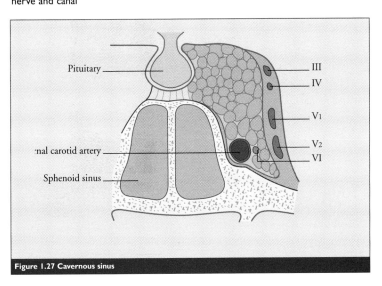

Figure 1.27 Cavernous sinus

Vertebrobasilar system
Vertebral artery branches within the skull
Meningeal
Posterior spinal
Anterior spinal
PICA — largest branch

Basilar artery branches
Pontine
Internal auditory
AICA
Superior cerebellar artery
Right and left posterior cerebral artery (thalamostriate, posterior
choroidal artery)

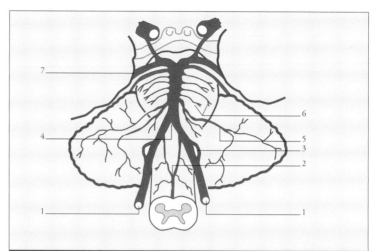

Figure 1.28 Anteroposterior view of the vertebrobasilar circulation (1) vertebral artery (2) anterior spinal artery (3) posterior inferior cerebellar artery (4) basilar artery (5) anterior inferior cerebellar artery (6) pontine perforating branches (7) posterior cerebral artery
Reprinted from Handbook of Neuroradiology: Brain & Skull (2nd Edition), Osborn & Tong, chapter 6, page 66: figure 6-1, 1996, by permission of Mosby.

Venous

Cerebral veins are characteristically thin walled, contain no valves and are in free communication

Can be divided into superficial and deep veins

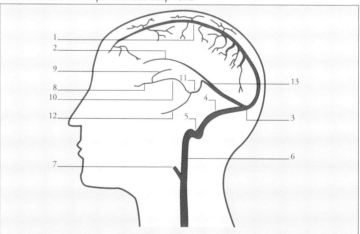

Figure 1.29 Lateral view of the cerebral venous system (1) superior sagittal sinus (2) inferior sagittal sinus (3) torcular herophili (4) transverse sinus (5) sigmoid sinus, jugular bulb (6) internal jugular vein (7) anterior branch of retromandibular vein (8) septal vein (9) thalamostriate vein (10) internal cerebral vein (11) vein of Galen (12) basal vein of Rosenthal (13) straight sinus
Reprinted from Handbook of Neuroradiology: Brain & Skull (2nd Edition), Osborn & Tong, chapter 7, page 76: figure 7-3, 1996, by permission of Mosby.

Superficial veins
Variable in position
Superior sagittal sinus more commonly drains into the right transverse sinus
Inferior sagittal sinus and great cerebral vein form the straight sinus which
drains into the left transverse sinus

Deep veins
More constant in appearance
Delineate the position of the lateral and third ventricles

Meninges
Three layers: pia mater, arachnoid and dura mater (inner to outer layers,
respectively)
Pia mater and dura mater are vascular; arachnoid is avascular

Dura mater
Firmly attached to the skull
Four septa (falx cerebri, falx cerebelli, tentorium cerebelli and
diaphragma sella)
Forms sheaths for the cranial nerves
Continuous with the sclera of the eye

1.3 The Vertebral Column

Forms the central axis of the skeleton
Provides support and protection
Made up of five parts, each having characteristic vertebrae

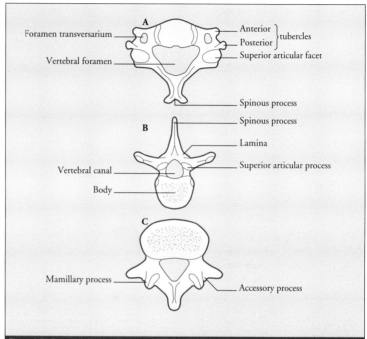

Figure 1.31 Essential characteristics of cervical, thoracic and lumbar vertebrae (A) a typical cervical vertebra, superior aspect (B) a typical thoracic vertebra, superior aspect (C) a typical lumbar vertebra, superior aspect
Reprinted from Essential Anatomy (4th Edition), Lumley, Craven & Aitken, chapter 3, page 44: figure 3.1, page 46: figure 3.4, page 46: figure 3.5, by permission of Churchill Livingstone.

Sacrum
There are five sacral vertebrae
Normally fused to form a single bone

Coccyx
Vestigial with no costal elements

Vertebral support
Vertebral disc
Secondary cartilaginous joint
A ring of fibrous tissue (annulus fibrosis)
Semi-liquid gelatinous centre (nucleus pulposis derived from the notochord)

Anterior longitudinal ligament
Extends from the anterior tubercle of the atlas to the front of the upper sacrum
Firmly attached to the periosteum of the vertebral bodies but not the discs

Posterior longitudinal ligament
Extends from the posterior surface of the axis (C2) to the sacral canal
Forms the tectorial membrane above the body of the axis
Firmly attached to the discs but not the vertebral bodies

Ligamenta flava
Join the contiguous borders of the adjacent laminae
Have a high content of elastic fibres (yellow)

Supraspinous ligaments
Join the tips of adjacent spinous processes
Strong bands of white fibrous tissue
Are replaced in the neck by the ligamentum nuchae

Interspinous ligaments
Unite the spinous processes along their adjacent borders
Fuse with the supraspinous ligaments
Are relatively weak

Intertransverse ligaments
Join the transverse processes along their adjacent borders
Form weak sheets of fibrous tissue

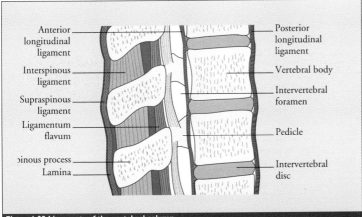

Figure 1.32 Ligaments of the vertebral column
Reprinted from Anatomy for Diagnostic Imaging, Ryan & McNichols, chapter 3, page 96: figure 3.13, 1994, by permission of WB Saunders Company.

Publisher's note: in Figure 1.32, the labels for the anterior and posterior longitudinal ligaments are reversed. The left label should read "Posterior longitudinal ligament" and the right label should read "Anterior longitudinal ligament"

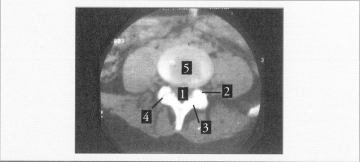

Figure 1.33 CT scan of lumbar spine (1) spinal canal (2) superior articular process (3) inferior articular process (4) facet joint (5) intervertebral disc

Spinal cord development
At birth, it ends at the lower border of L3
In adult life, it lies between T12 and L3
Dural sac extends to S3
Widest at C5 and T12 segmental levels
Occupies no more than 80% of the transverse diameter of the dural space
Cervical nerve roots exit above the corresponding vertebral bodies
Thoracic, lumbar and sacral roots exit below their corresponding vertebral bodies

Blood supply
Single anterior spinal artery
Paired posterior spinal arteries
Multiple radicular arteries

Artery of Adamckiewicz is a large radicular artery — 60% on the left side and 75% between T9 and T12
Venous drainage follows the arterial pattern

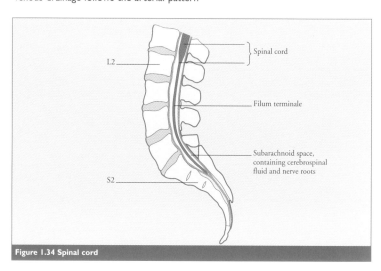

Figure 1.34 Spinal cord

1.4 The Head and Neck

Skull

Flat bones of the neurocranium and facial skeleton ossify in membrane: maxilla, mandible, squamous portion of the occiput, frontal, parietal and occipital bone
Bones of the skull base ossify in cartilage: sphenoid, mastoid, petrous temple

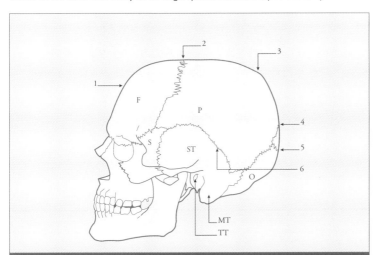

Figure 1.41 Lateral view of adult skull indicating calvarial bones and sutures
Bones (F) frontal bone (P) parietal bone (O) occipital bone (ST) squamous portion of temporal bone (MT) mastoid portion of temporal bone (TT) tympanic portion of temporal bone (S) sphenoid bone
Sutures (1) metopic suture (2) coronal suture (3) sagittal suture (4) lambdoid suture (5) mendosal suture (6) squamosal suture

Bony landmarks

Bregma — junction of the coronal and sagittal sutures
Lambda — junction of the sagittal and lamboid sutures
Pterion — 'H' junction of the great wing of the sphenoid, frontal, parietal and squamous part of the temple bone (the surface marker of the middle meningeal artery)
Asterion — junction of the temporal, occipital and parietal bone
Sphenoccipital synchondrosis — articulation between the occipital and sphenoid bone joined by a cartilaginous joint (fusion at 25 years and may mimic a fracture)

Accessory sutures

Metopic suture
Divides the frontal bone
Normally disappears by the age of 2 years
10% persist into adult life and are associated with an absence of the frontal sinus

Mendosal suture
Found entirely within the occipital bone

Skull foramina

There are six major foramina

Two in each of the sphenoid, petrous temporal and occipital bone

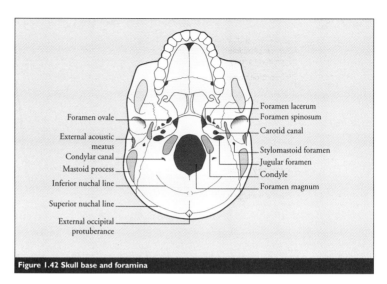

Foramen ovale

External acoustic meatus

Condylar canal

Mastoid process

Inferior nuchal line

Superior nuchal line

External occipital protuberance

Foramen lacerum

Foramen spinosum

Carotid canal

Stylomastoid foramen

Jugular foramen

Condyle

Foramen magnum

Figure 1.42 Skull base and foramina

Jugular foramen

Interosseous membrane passing between the occipital and petrous temporal bones

Two compartments

Internal auditory meatus

Transmits the VII and VIII nerves

Four separate compartments

Foramen magnum

Transmits the medulla oblongata, spinal arteries and veins, the cervical roots of the XI nerve and the apical ligament

Dimensions: anteroposterior 3.2-3.67 cm, transverse 2.5-3.4 cm

Hypoglossal canal

Transmits the XII nerve

Anterior to the occipital condyle

Foramina	Transmits	Observed on	Special notes
Optic canal	II	Special views	6-7 mm diameter ≤1 mm difference between sides
Superior orbital fissure	V₁ III, IV, VI Superior ophthalmic vein Branch of middle meningeal artery	OF	Lateral to optic canal
Inferior orbital fissure	Infraorbital nerve anatomy	20° OF	Runs between pterygopalatine fossa (posteriorly) and infratemporal fossa (anteriorly)
Foramen rotundum	V₂	20° OF	Leads to pterygopalatine fossa
Foramen ovale	V₃ Accessory meningeal artery	SMV	Leads to infratemporal fossa
Foramen spinosum	Middle meningeal artery	SMV	Leads to infratemporal fossa
Foramen lacerum		SMV	
Carotid canal	Internal carotid artery	SMV	
Internal auditory meatus		OF Townes SMV	
Jugular foramen	IX, X, XI Internal jugular vein Inferior petrosal sinus	Special views	
Hypoglossal canal	XII	1/2 SMV Special views	
Foramen magnum	Spinal cord Vertebral artery and vein Anterior spinal arteries Spinal venous plexus Spinal root XI	SMV	
Pituitary fossa		20° OF, Townes, SMV, lateral	
Zygoma		OM, Townes, SMV	
Orbital margin and floor		20° OF, 30° OM	
Paranasal sinuses		20° OF, OM Open mouth (sphenoid) Lateral, SMV, 30° OM	
SMV			
Mandible		20° OF, 30° OM Lateral, OPG	

OF = Occipitofrontal
OM = Occipitomental
OPG = Orthopantomogram
SMV = Submentovertex

Table 1.41 Skull radiographics

The orbit

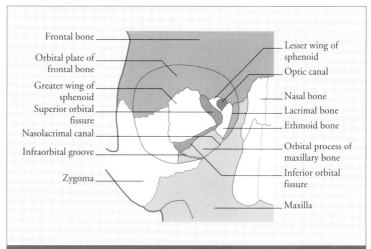

Frontal bone

Orbital plate of frontal bone

Greater wing of sphenoid

Superior orbital fissure

Nasolacrimal canal

Infraorbital groove

Zygoma

Lesser wing of sphenoid

Optic canal

Nasal bone

Lacrimal bone

Ethmoid bone

Orbital process of maxillary bone

Inferior orbital fissure

Maxilla

Figure 1.43 Bony orbit
Reprinted from Anatomy for Diagnostic Imaging, Ryan & McNichols, chapter 1, page 11: figure 1.9, 1994, by permission of WB Saunders Company.

Optic foramen
Transmits the optic nerve and ophthalmic artery (branch of the internal carotid artery)
Formed at the apex of the orbit
Positioned medially to the orbital fissures
Maximal diameter is 7 mm
Pathological if there is >1 mm difference between the sides

Superior orbital fissure
Situated between the greater and lesser wings of the sphenoid
Asymmetrical

Inferior orbital fissure
Situated between the greater wing of the sphenoid and the roof of the maxillary antrum
Communicates with the sphenopalatine, pterygopalatine and infratemporal fossae

Fossae of the skull
Infratemporal fossa

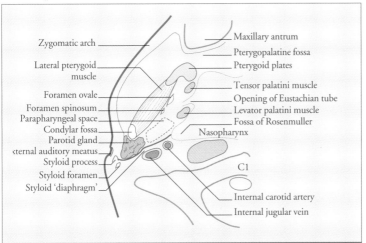

Zygomatic arch

Lateral pterygoid muscle

Foramen ovale

Foramen spinosum

Parapharyngeal space

Condylar fossa

Parotid gland

External auditory meatus

Styloid process

Styloid foramen

Styloid 'diaphragm'

Maxillary antrum

Pterygopalatine fossa

Pterygoid plates

Tensor palatini muscle

Opening of Eustachian tube

Levator palatini muscle

Fossa of Rosenmuller

Nasopharynx

C1

Internal carotid artery

Internal jugular vein

Figure 1.44 Infratemporal fossa: axial section
Reprinted from Anatomy for Diagnostic Imaging, Ryan & McNichols, chapter 1, page 29: figure 1.30, 1994, by permission of WB Saunders Company.

Boundaries
Ramus of the mandible
Zygomatic arch and temporalis muscle
Lateral wall of the pharynx and maxilla
Temporal surface of the greater wing of the sphenoid

Communicates with
Inferior orbital fissure
Pterygopalatine fissure
Temporal fossa

Contents
Pterygoid and temporalis muscles
Maxillary and mandibular divisions of the trigeminal nerve (plus otic ganglion)
Pterygoid venous plexus

Pterygopalatine fossa
Small pyramidal space
Inferior to the apex of the orbit

Anterior	Maxilla
Posterior	Pterygoid fossa of the sphenoid bone
Medial	Palatine bone
Lateral	Opens into the infratemporal fossa
Roof	Greater wing of the sphenoid bone (incomplete)

Table 1.42 Boundaries of the pterygopalatine fossa

Communicates with
Orbit via the inferior orbital fissure
Middle cranial fossa via the foramen rotundum
Infratemporal fossa
Nose via the sphenopalatine foramen
Mouth via the greater and lesser palatine foramina

Contents
Maxillary division of the trigeminal nerve
Five branches of the internal maxillary artery (posterior superior alveolar,
greater palatine, sphenopalatine, inferior orbital, pharyngeal)
Pterygopalatine ganglion (parasympathetic)
(Vidian artery and nerve)

Mandible
Temporomandibular joint

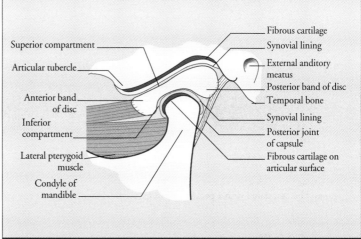

Figure 1.45 Temporomandibular joint
Reprinted from Anatomy for Diagnostic Imaging, Ryan & McNichols, chapter 1, page 14: figure 1.13, 1994, by
permission of WB Saunders Company.

Synovial hinge joint between the condyle of the mandible and the mandibular fossa
Dislocation is prevented by the articular tubercle of the temporal bone
The joint is separated into superior and inferior compartments by a
fibrocartilaginous articular disc
Disc is attached to the lateral pterygoid muscle
On opening, rotational movement occurs in the inferior compartment and forward
movement in the superior compartment

Sphenomandibular ligament
Attached to the sphenoid bone and the lingula on the medial surface of the ramus
of the mandible

Stylomandibular ligament

Attached to the styloid process and the posterior border of the angle of the mandible

Nasal cavity and paranasal sinuses

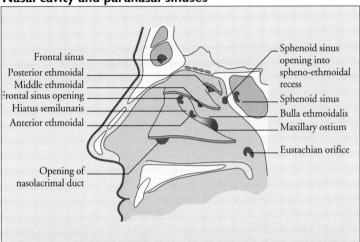

Frontal sinus
Posterior ethmoidal
Middle ethmoidal
Frontal sinus opening
Hiatus semilunaris
Anterior ethmoidal

Sphenoid sinus opening into spheno-ethmoidal recess
Sphenoid sinus
Bulla ethmoidalis
Maxillary ostium

Eustachian orifice

Opening of nasolacrimal duct

Figure 1.46 The lateral wall of the right nasal cavity — the conchae have been partially removed to show structures that drain into the nose
Reprinted from Clinical Anatomy, Ellis, pt. 5, The Head and Neck, page 342: figure 225, 1997, by permission of Blackwell Science Ltd.

Frontal sinus

Only sinus present at birth
Not observed on plain films until approximately 2 years of age
Full size attained at approximately 14 years of age
Absence may be associated with a persistent metopic suture

Ethmoidal cells

Appear at 2 years of age
Fully developed by 14 years of age
Anterior and middle cells open into the middle meatus
Posterior cells open into the superior meatus

Sphenoid sinus

Appears at approximately 3 years of age
Normally has a septum

Maxillary sinus

Appears just after birth
Fully developed by 6 years of age

Lacrimal apparatus

Lacrimal gland

Lies in a hollow in the upper lateral part of the front of the orbit
Supplied by parasympathetic fibres via the pterygopalatine ganglion

Nasolacrimal duct

Tears drain via two lacrimal canaliculi into the duct
3 cm in length with three constrictions
Empties into the lateral wall of the nose via the inferior meatus

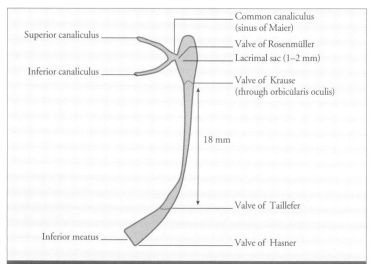

Superior canaliculus

Inferior canaliculus

Common canaliculus (sinus of Maier)

Valve of Rosenmüller

Lacrimal sac (1–2 mm)

Valve of Krause (through orbicularis oculis)

18 mm

Valve of Taillefer

Inferior meatus

Valve of Hasner

Figure 1.47 Nasolacrimal duct
Reprinted from Aids to Part I FRCR, Hornsby & Winter, chapter 2, page 57: figure 31, 1988, by permission of Churchill Livingstone.

Ear

External meatus

3.5 cm long
Outer third is cartilaginous and the inner two-thirds are bony

Eustachian tube

Runs anteromedial and is 3.5 cm long
Inner third is bony and the outer two-thirds are cartilaginous
Opens into the nasopharynx with the taurus tubarus (cartilaginous elevation) posteriorly

Tegmen tympani

1 cm long
Separates the middle ear from the middle cranial fossa

Middle ear

Three auditory ossicles: malleus, incus and stapes (connected to the oval window)

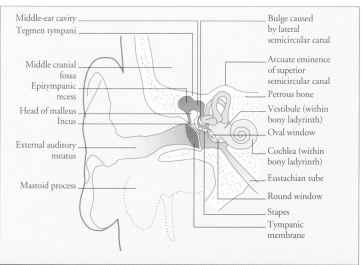

Figure 1.48 Ear — coronal section showing outer, middle and inner ear
Reprinted from Anatomy for Diagnostic Imaging, Ryan & McNichols, chapter 1, page 24: figure 1.25, 1994, by permission of WB Saunders Company.

Inner ear

Cochlear consists of 2³/₄ turns

Arcuate eminence of the petrous temporal bone is formed by the superior semicircular canal

Membranous labyrinth consists of the saccula, utricle, semicircular canals and cochlear duct

Internal meatus

1 cm long

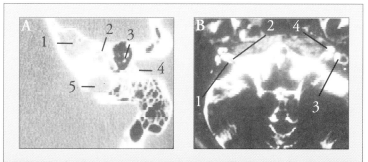

Figure 1.49A Axial CT scan of the middle ear (1) petrous apex (2) cochlea (3) incudo-malleolar joint (4) external auditory meatus (5) jugular bulb
Figure 1.49B MRI scan of the internal auditory meatus (1) vestibulocochlear nerve (2) facial nerve (3) vestibule (4) cochlea

Salivary glands

Parotid gland

Predominantly a serous gland

Parotid (Stensen's) duct

Superficial to masseter
Pierces buccinator
Opens opposite the second upper molar

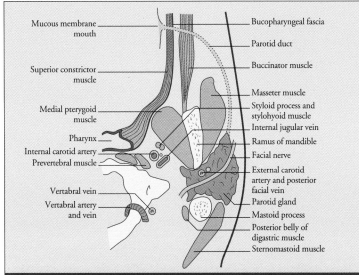

Figure 1.410 Relations of the parotid gland
Reprinted from Anatomy for Diagnostic Imaging, Ryan & McNichols, chapter 1, page 18: figure 1.18 (B), 1994, by permission of WB Saunders Company.

Submandibular gland

Predominantly a mucous-secreting gland
Situated in the submandibular triangle, with superficial and deep portions around mylohyoid
Submandibular (Wharton's) duct opens in the floor of the mouth, adjacent to the frenulum

Pharynx

Fibromuscular tube extending from the base of the skull to the level of C6 (level of cricopharyngeus)
Only pierced by the eustachian tube
Consists of three constrictor muscles (superior, middle, inferior) and three other muscles (cricopharyngeus, palatopharyngeus, stylopharyngeus)
Inferior constrictor can be divided into oblique and transverse components
The gap between is known as Killean's dehiscence — the area in which pharyngeal pouches are formed

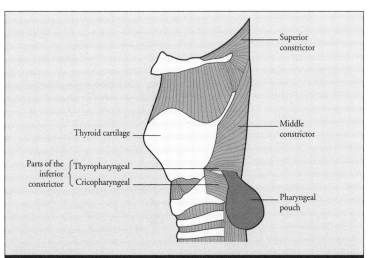

Superior constrictor

Middle constrictor

Thyroid cartilage

Parts of the inferior constrictor { Thyropharyngeal
Cricopharyngeal

Pharyngeal pouch

Figure 1.411 A pharyngeal pouch emerging between the two components of the inferior constrictor muscle
Reprinted from Clinical Anatomy, Ellis, pt. 5, The Head and Neck, page 305: figure 204, 1997, by permission of Blackwell Science Ltd.

Piriform fossae

Paired recesses on either side of the laryngeal orifice
Lie between the aryepiglottic membrane medially and the laminae of the thyroid cartilage laterally
Broad above and narrow below

Soft tissue of neck

Extends from the skull base to cricopharyngeus
Dimensions:
C1-C4   ≤7 mm
C4-C6   ≤21 mm

Larynx

Respiratory passage between the laryngopharynx and the trachea
Allows phonation and protects the respiratory airway
Lies between the level of C3 and C6
Consists of three single and three paired cartilages
Single cartilages are the epiglottis (fibrocartilage; FC), thyroid (hyaline cartilage; H) and cricohyoid (H)
Paired cartilages are the arytenoids (H), cuneiform (FC) and corniculate (FC)
Laryngeal prominence — 90° in males and 120° in females

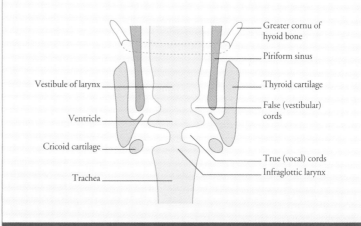

Figure 1.412 Coronal section of the larynx
Reprinted from Anatomy for Diagnostic Imaging, Ryan & McNichols, chapter 1, page 32: figure 1.33 (B), 1994, by permission of WB Saunders Company.

Cricoid cartilage

Flat and wide to posterior
Narrow anterior arch

Appearance on MRI

Cartilage has a high signal (fatty marrow)
False cords have a high signal
True cords (ligamentous) have a low signal

Vocal cord attachments

Anterior — thyrocartilage
Posterior — arytenoid cartilages

Muscles

All are adductors except for the posterior cricoarytenoid (abductor)
All the muscles are supplied by the recurrent laryngeal nerve except for the cricothyroid (external laryngeal nerve)

Thyroid gland
Enclosed within the pretracheal fascia
Consists of two lobes connected via a median isthmus
Lobes extend from C5 to T1

Arterial supply
Superior thyroid artery (external carotid artery)
Inferior thyroid artery (thyrocervical trunk — subclavian artery)

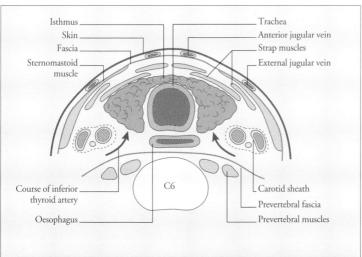

Figure 1.413 Transverse section through the neck
Reprinted from Anatomy for Diagnostic Imaging, Ryan & McNichols, chapter 1, page 36: figure 1.36(B), 1994, by permission of WB Saunders Company.

Venous drainage
Superior and middle thyroid veins (drain to the internal jugular veins)
Inferior thyroid veins (drain to the brachiocephalic veins)

Parathyroid gland
Normally four glands
Superior glands arise from the fourth pouch and have a constant position
Inferior glands arise from the third pouch and have a variable position
Ultrasound homogeneously hypoechoic

Vascular supply of the head and neck

Subclavian artery

Divided into three parts by scalenus anterior and terminates at the outer border of the first rib (see diagram)

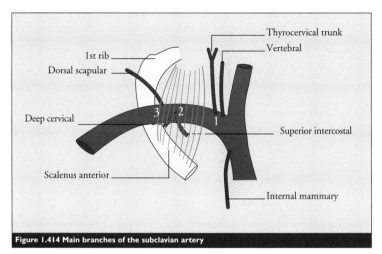

Figure 1.414 Main branches of the subclavian artery

Common carotid artery

Arises on the right from the brachiocephalic artery and on the left directly from the aortic arch

At the level of the upper border of the thyroid cartilage (C4) it divides into the external and internal carotid arteries

External carotid artery initially lies anteriorly and medial to the internal carotid artery

At the level of C2 it comes to lie lateral

The following structures pass between the external and internal carotid arteries:

1. glossopharyngeal nerve (IX)
2. stylopharyngeus
3. pharyngeal branch of the vagus nerve (X)

Internal carotid artery has no significant branches within the neck

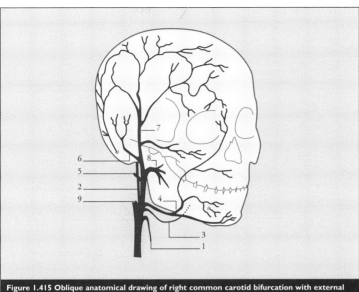

Figure 1.415 Oblique anatomical drawing of right common carotid bifurcation with external carotid artery and major branches (1) superior thyroid (2) ascending pharyngeal (3) lingual (4) facial (5) occipital (6) posterior auricular (7) superficial temporal (8) maxillary (9) internal carotid
Reprinted from Handbook of Neuroradiology: Brain & Skull (2nd Edition), Osborn & Tong, chapter 3, page 33: figure 3-2, 1996, by permission of Mosby.

Branches of the external carotid artery
Maxillary artery
Arises from the external carotid artery within the parotid gland
Posterior relation of the neck of the mandible
Divided into three portions by its relation with the lateral pterygoid muscle

Middle meningeal artery
Arises from the first part of the maxillary artery
Passes intracranially via the foramen spinosum within the greater wing of the sphenoid
Surface marking is the pterion

Venous drainage
Via the internal and external jugular vein
Internal jugular vein — a continuation of the sigmoid and inferior petrosal sinuses and is related initially posterior then laterally to the internal carotid artery
External jugular vein — lies within the superficial tissues of the neck and drains into the subclavian vein

1.5 The Thorax

Ribs

12 pairs — 7 true, 3 false and 2 floating

Atypical ribs

1st — single costovertebral joint (articulates only with T1)
2nd — site of attachment for second head of scalenus anterior
10th-12th ribs have a single articular facet at their head

Radiological variations

Upper ribs

Commonly show fusion, bifurcation, hyperplasia
Costochondral calcification is marginal in males and central in females

Cervical ribs

Present in 1.5% of the population
50% are bilateral
More common in females
Can be made of fibrous bands/bone

Sternum

Consists of the manubrium, body and xiphoid process

Manubrium

Level T3/T4
Articulates with the clavicle and 1^1/2 costochondral junctions

Sternal angle

Level T4/T5 disc space
Secondary cartilaginous joint

Body

Level T5/T9
Made of four sternebrae

Xiphoid process

Cartilaginous
Separate, fuses from 40 years onwards

	Primary centres	**Secondary centres**
Ribs	Angle of the rib 8th week *in utero*	Head/tubercle 15 years (fusion at 25 years)
Sternum	Superior to inferior 5-9th month *in utero*	Fusion inferior to superior 15-20 years (except xiphoid process)
Clavicle	Shaft 5-6th week *in utero*	Sternal end 18-20 years (fusion at 25 years)

Table 1.51 Ossification centres in the thorax

Companion shadows
Soft-tissue shadows seen on plain radiographs
Found in association with the inferior surface of:
1. clavicles
2. upper ribs
3. lower ribs (laterally)

Soft-tissue shadows
Nipple
Typically well defined laterally and poorly defined medially
Confirm using nipple markers

Axilla
Anterior (oblique orientation) and posterior (vertical orientation) folds

Muscles
Pectoralis major
Sternocleidomastoid

Thymus
Extends from the thyroid to the level of the fourth costal cartilage
Reaches maximum size by the second decade
Can be seen in neonates, infants and young children on a posterior-anterior (PA) chest film
Typically sail shaped, wavy outline, changes shape with respiration

Pleura
Two layers of visceral and parietal
Visceral pleura extends into the fissures
Both layers join at the hilum to form the pulmonary ligament

Fissures
Horizontal (minor)
Extends from the sixth rib laterally
Does not extend beyond the lobar pulmonary artery medially
May only be seen in a very small segment
Visible on the PA and lateral chest films

Oblique (major)
Extends from T4 posteriorly, curving downwards to the diaphragm inferiorly
Upper portion faces forward and laterally
Lower portion faces posteriorly and laterally (propeller shaped)
To differentiate between sides, the left fissure characteristically:
1. is more vertical
2. has a more posterior junction with the diaphragm
3. does not intersect with the minor fissure

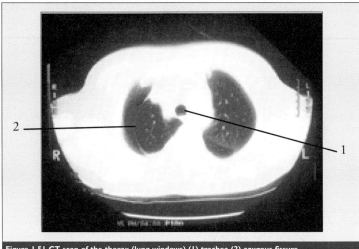

Figure 1.51 CT scan of the thorax (lung windows) (1) trachea (2) azygous fissure

Accessory fissures
Azygos fissure
Present in 0.5-1% of the population
Four layers surrounding the azygos vein
Can be left sided, enclosing the hemiazygos vein

Inferior accessory fissure
Present in 5-10% of the population
Most commonly right sided
Separates the medial basal segment from the other basal segments

Superior accessory fissure
Present in 5% of the population
Apical segment of the lower lobe
Most commonly right sided

Left horizontal fissure
Present in 1% of the population
Separates the lingula from the upper lobe

Diaphragm
Outline
Arcuate ligaments — median, medial, lateral
Well-defined costophrenic (CP) angle
Poorly defined cardiophrenic angle due to fat within the oblique fissure

Normal variants
Muscle slips
Anteromedial hump (right)
Rounded CP angle in the young

Height
In 94% of the population, right>left by 2.5 cm
In 5% of the population, left>right

Movement
Up to 9 cm on deep respiration

Nerve supply
Phrenic nerve (C3-C5)

Crura
Right crus — extends from LI to L3
Left crus — extends from LI to L2

Orientation of the domes of the diaphragm on the lateral chest X-ray
Gastric bubble below the left hemi-diaphragm
Fissure identification
Left hemi-diaphragm obscured by the base of the heart
Right hemi-diaphragm passes through the heart

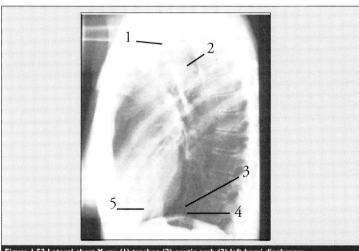

Figure 1.52 Lateral chest X-ray (1) trachea (2) aortic arch (3) left hemi-diaphragm (4) gastric bubble (5) right hemi-diaphragm

Diaphragmatic openings
T8 — inferior vena cava (IVC), right phrenic nerve
T10 — oesophagus, anterior and posterior vagal trunks, left gastric artery and vein
T12 — aorta, thoracic duct, azygos and hemiazygos veins

Mediastinum markings

Line — air outlining a soft-tissue structure
Stripe — air outlining either side of a structure

Anterior junctional line

Anterior point of contact between the right and left pleural lines
Below the level of the suprasternal notch

Posterior junctional line

Apposition of the two lungs posteriorly
Above the sternal notch to the level of the arch of the aorta

Azygo-oesophageal line

Inverted 'J' shape
Corresponds to the arch of the azygos vein

Paratracheal line

5 mm
Right paratracheal stripe extends from the azygos vein to the innominate artery
Widened in malignancy, mediastinitis, pleural effusion, nodal disease
No left paratracheal line due to the presence of the aorta

Paraspinal lines

Right (2 mm) — parallel to the vertebrae
Left (<1 cm) — affected by the aorta

Aorto-pulmonary window

Between the aortic arch and the left pulmonary artery (LPA)
Contents: ligamentum arteriosum, fat, ductus node, left recurrent laryngeal nerve, left vagus nerve, left bronchial artery

Retrosternal line

<2 mm
Observed in the lateral view
Straight appearance

Parasternal line

<5 mm
Wavy outline
Observed in the lateral view
Increases in width with the presence of internal mammary nodes

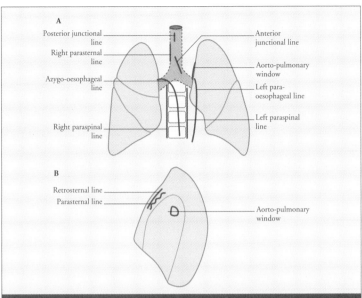

A

Posterior junctional line
Right parasternal line
Azygo-oesophageal line
Right paraspinal line

Anterior junctional line
Aorto-pulmonary window
Left para-oesophageal line
Left paraspinal line

B

Retrosternal line
Parasternal line
Aorto-pulmonary window

Figure 1.53 Mediastinal contours (A) anterior view (B) lateral view

Right heart border	Left heart border
Right subclavian vein	Left subclavian artery
	Aortic knuckle
	Main pulmonary artery
Superior vena cava	Left atrial appendage
Right atrium	Left ventricle

Table 1.52 Mediastinal silhouette

Trachea

Extends from the cricoid cartilage (C6) to the level of the carina (T4)
10-11 cm long with 15-20 rings
Descends to the right due to the presence of the aortic arch
Carinal angle 55-80°
Diameter is 2.5 cm in males and 2.1 cm in females

Bronchi

Compared with the left main stem bronchus, the right main stem bronchus is:
1. shorter
2. wider
3. more vertical
4. lower than the left in 97% of individuals and equal in 3%

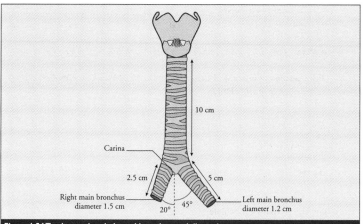

Figure 1.54 Trachea and main bronchi — sizes and dimensions

10 cm

Carina

2.5 cm   5 cm

Right main bronchus
diameter 1.5 cm

20°   45°

Left main bronchus
diameter 1.2 cm

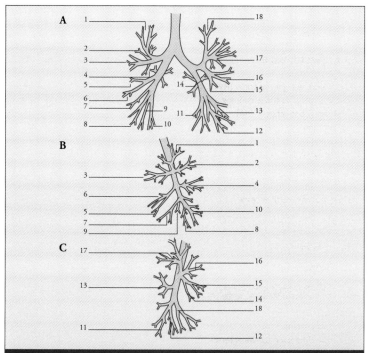

Figure 1.55 Bronchopulmonary segments (A) anteroposterior view **(B)** lateral view of right bronchial tree **(C)** lateral view of left bronchial tree; **(1)** apical segment **(2)** posterior segment **(3)** anterior segment **(4)** superior segment **(5)** lateral segment **(6)** medial segment **(7)** anterior basal segment **(8)** lateral basal segment **(9)** posterior segment **(10)** medial basal segment **(11)** posterior basal segment **(12)** lateral basal segment **(13)** anterior medial basal segment **(14)** superior segment **(15)** inferior segment (lingula) **(16)** superior segment (lingula) **(17)** anterior segment **(18)** apicoposterior segment

Bronchopulmonary segments

Within the right middle lobe, the right lateral segment bronchus arises superior to the medial segment bronchus

Apical segment of the right lower lobe arises at the same level as the middle lobe bronchus

Order of the segmental bronchi of the lower lobe from lateral to medial-frontal view is ALPM, oblique view is PMLA

Minor airways

Conductive

Finish at the level of the terminal bronchiole

<2 mm in diameter

Loose cilia, cartilage and goblet cells

Acinous

Supplied by the terminal bronchiole

Approximately 6 mm in diameter

Alveoli

Type 1/type 2 pneumocytes

350×10^6 in the adult lung

Lung vasculature

Pulmonary artery

Arises from the right ventricle (RV)

Passes posterior to the ascending aorta and superior vena cava (SVC); anterior to the rightmain bronchus (RMB)

The main pulmonary artery divides in the arch of the aorta, anterior to the left main bronchus (LMB)

Diameter is 16 mm in males and 15 mm in females

Right pulmonary artery	Left pulmonary artery
Longer	Shorter
Anterior to RMB	Posterior to LMB
Divides in the hilum of the lung	Attached to the aorta via the ligamentum arteriosum

Table 1.53 Features of the right versus left pulmonary artery

Pulmonary veins

Anterior and inferior to the arteries

Hilar point

Intersection of the upper-lobe pulmonary vein and the descending pulmonary artery

Right side is lower than the left (due to the LPA arching over the LMB)

Forms an angle of approximately 120°

Bronchial arteries

Arise from the aorta at the T5/T6 level
Usually one right artery and two left arteries
In less than 10% of cases, bronchial arteries may arise from the subclavian or internal thoracic artery

Heart

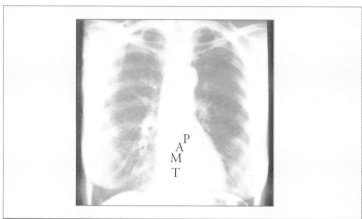

Figure 1.56 Chest X-ray of heart with valves marked (P) pulmonary valve (A) aortic valve (M) mitral valve (T) tricuspid valve

Coronary arteries

Arise from the ascending aorta and supply the myocardium

Right coronary artery

Originates from the right aortic sinus
Passes between the pulmonary trunk and right auricle to enter the atrioventricular (AV) sulcus
Runs along the inferior surface of the heart
90% of individuals have dominance of the right coronary artery
Supplies the right atrium (RA), sinoatrial (SA) node (60%), RV, interventricular septum and AV node (80%)
Branches — right marginal, posterior interventricular

Left coronary artery

Arises from the left posterior aortic sinus
Passes posterior to the pulmonary trunk and anterior to the left auricle
Forms the anterior interventricular and circumflex arteries
Supplies the left atrium (LA), left ventricle (LV), anterior interventricular septum, SA node (40%) and AV node (20%)

Coronary veins
Follow the arteries

Coronary sinus
Drains into the back of the RA and receives:
1. the great cardiac vein (anterior interventricular groove)
2. the middle cardiac vein (posterior interventricular groove)
3. small cardiac veins (coronary sulcus)

Anterior cardiac veins
From the RV, drain directly into the RA

Venae cordis minimae
From the RA, drain directly into the wall of the RA

Great vessels
Ascending aorta
Arises at the vestibule of the LV (T6)
Becomes the aortic arch at the level of the manubriosternal joint (T4)
Enclosed in both fibrous and serous pericardium

Anterior	Right auricle, infundibulum, pulmonary trunk
Posterior	LA, right pulmonary artery, RMB
Left	Pulmonary trunk, left auricle
Right	SVC, RA

Table 1.54 Relations of the ascending aorta

Aortic arch
Passes over the LMB
The highest point is the midpoint of the manubrium sternae (T2)
Three main branches:
1. brachiocephalic artery
2. left common carotid artery
3. left subclavian artery

Anterior	Left phrenic nerve, left vagus, left superior intercostal vein
Posterior	Trachea, left recurrent laryngeal nerve, oesophagus, thoracic duct
Inferior	Pulmonary bifurcation, LMB, ligamentum arteriosum, left recurrent laryngeal nerve
Lateral	Left lung and pleura

Table 1.55 Relations of the aortic arch

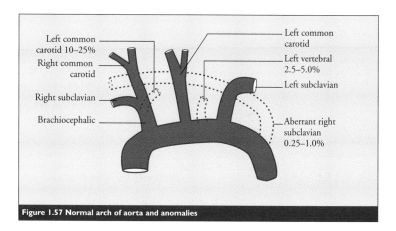

Figure 1.57 Normal arch of aorta and anomalies

Normal variants
Left common carotid artery — 10-25% are of brachiocephalic origin
Left vertebral artery — 2.5-5% arise directly from the aortic arch
Aberrant right subclavian artery — in 0.25-1% of individuals, this arises distal to the left subclavian artery; can result in dysphagia as it creates a posterior indentation on the oesophagus

Thoracic (descending) aorta
Arises as a continuation of the aortic arch
Commences to the left of the body of T4
Ends as it passes into the abdomen at T12
Grooves the left side of the bodies of T4-T6
Inclines medially to come to lie in the midline of T8-T12

Inferior	Hilum of the left lung, LMB, pericardium, LA, oesophagus
Posterior	Necks of the 5th and 6th ribs, sympathetic chain, hemiazygos veins
Right	Right pleura, right lung, thoracic duct Oesophagus initially to the right but becomes to lie anterior and slightly to the left
Left	Left pleura, left lung

Table 1.56 Relations of the thoracic aorta

SVC

Arises as a result of the union of the right and left brachiocephalic veins, behind the first costochondral cartilage
Receives the azygos vein on its posterior surface at the level of T4
Enters the RA at the level of T5

Inferior	Right atrial appendage
Posterior	Right pulmonary artery, azygos vein, trachea
Laterally	Right phrenic nerve, right lung

Table 1.57 Relations of the superior vena cava

Azygos venous system

Continuation of the ascending lumbar veins and posterior drainage of the thoracic wall
Single system on the right
Two systems on the left — hemiazygos and accessory hemiazygos

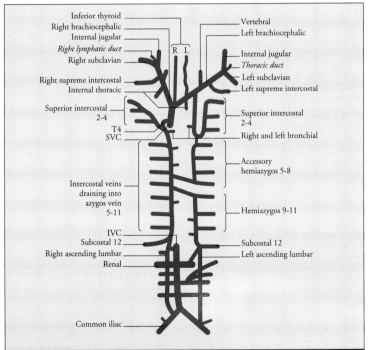

Figure 1.58 Superior vena cava and azygous veins; accessory hemiazygos crosses to azygos at T7 and hemiazygos at T8; each crosses behind the thoracic aorta, oesophagus and thoracic duct (lymphatic drainage marked in italics)

Azygos vein

Arises from the confluence of the right ascending lumbar and right subcostal vein

Passes through the aortic opening of the diaphragm at the level of T12 (posterior to the oesophagus and to the right of the aorta)

Runs anterior over the hilum of the right lung (lateral to the oesophagus, trachea and

right vagus nerve)

Enters the SVC at T4

Tributaries

The eight lower right posterior intercostal veins

Right superior intercostal vein

Bronchial veins

Oesophageal veins

The two hemiazygos veins

Hemiazygos vein

Arises from the confluence of the left ascending lumbar vein and left subcostal vein

Often a tributary of the left renal vein

Ascends through the aortic opening of the diaphragm (to the left of the thoracic vertebra)

At T9 crosses posteriorly (to the aorta, oesophagus and thoracic duct) to enter the azygos vein at T8

Drains the four lower left posterior intercostal veins (9-12)

Accessory hemiazygos vein

Drains the 5th-8th left posterior intercostal veins

Runs inferiorly on the left side of the vertebral bodies to T8

Crosses posteriorly to enter the azygos vein at T7

Tributaries from the bronchial and mid-oesophageal veins

Superior intercostal vein

Drains the 2nd-4th intercostal veins

Enters the inferior aspect of the brachiocephalic vein

May be seen as a 'nipple' on the anteroposterior view of the aortic arch

Supreme intercostal veins

Drain the 1st intercostal space

Drain into their respective brachiocephalic veins

Nerves (relations)

Right vagus

Runs on the anterior aspect of scalenus anterior in the neck
Anterior to the right subclavian artery
Passes between the trachea and the azygos vein, lateral to the oesophagus
Forms the posterior vagal trunk within the abdomen, passing through the diaphragm
at the level of T10

Left vagus

Runs anterior to scalenus anterior in the neck
Passes anterior to the thoracic duct and oesophagus
Posterior to the left brachiocephalic vein, descending aorta and LA
Passes through the diaphragm at the level of T10, forming the anterior vagal trunk

Right phrenic nerve

Anterior to scalenus anterior and posterior to the right subclavian vein
Runs lateral to the SVC and fibrous pericardium
Passes anterior to the hilum of the lung
Passes through the diaphragm at the level of T8 with the IVC

Left phrenic nerve

Passes posterior to the thoracic duct and the origin of the left brachiocephalic vein
Runs lateral to the arch of the aorta
Anterior to the hilum of the lung
Pierces but does not pass through the diaphragm

Thoracic duct (see Abdomen)

1.6 The Abdomen

Abdominal wall
Three-muscle wall layer — external oblique, internal oblique and transversus abdominus
Layers are separated by properitoneal fat, which is visible on a plain abdominal film

Umbilical ligaments
Median — fibrous remnant of the urachus
Medial — obliterated umbilical arteries
Lateral — contains the inferior epigastric artery

Peritoneum
Serous membrane lining the abdominal and pelvic cavities
All organs lie outside the peritoneum, but if they invaginate, they can be entirely covered by the peritoneum
Double folds of peritoneum are termed mesenteries/ligaments
Normal peritoneum is not visible on any imaging modality

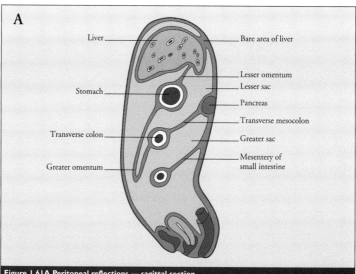

A

Liver
Bare area of liver
Lesser omentum
Lesser sac
Stomach
Pancreas
Transverse mesocolon
Transverse colon
Greater sac
Greater omentum
Mesentery of small intestine

Figure 1.61A Peritoneal reflections — sagittal section
Reprinted from Clinical Anatomy, Ellis, pt. 2, The Abdomen and Pelvis, page 70: figure 47, 1997, by permission of Blackwell Science Ltd.

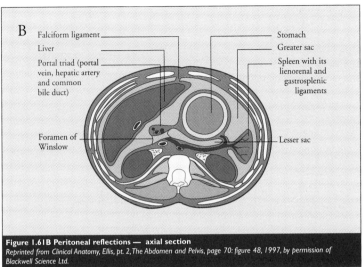

B
Falciform ligament
Liver
Portal triad (portal vein, hepatic artery and common bile duct)
Foramen of Winslow

Stomach
Greater sac
Spleen with its lienorenal and gastrosplenic ligaments
Lesser sac

Figure 1.61B Peritoneal reflections — axial section
Reprinted from Clinical Anatomy, Ellis, pt. 2, The Abdomen and Pelvis, page 70: figure 48, 1997, by permission of Blackwell Science Ltd.

The peritoneal compartment can be divided along the line of the transverse mesocolon into supra- and infracolic spaces
The infracolic space can be further subdivided into right and left along the line of the mesentery of the small bowel

Subphrenic spaces

Lie between the diaphragm and liver on either side of the falciform ligament

Right subhepatic space (hepatorenal pouch of Morrison)

Lies between the liver and right kidney
The most dependent part of the abdominal cavity when the patient is supine

Left subhepatic space

Lesser sac
Communicates with the right subhepatic space through the epiploic foramen

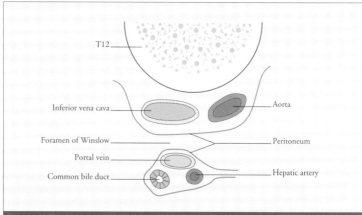

Figure 1.62 The foramen of Winslow in transverse section
Reprinted from Clinical Anatomy, Ellis, pt. 2, The Abdomen and Pelvis, page 72: figure 49, 1997, by permission of Blackwell Science Ltd.

Boundaries of the epiploic foramen

Anterior — portal vein, common bile duct and hepatic artery
Posterior — inferior vena cava (IVC)
Superior — caudate lobe of the liver
Inferior — first part of the duodenum

Oesophagus

Extends from the level of the cricoid cartilage (C6) to the cardia
Total length 25 cm

Anatomical constrictions

Cricopharyngeus
Left main bronchus
Cardia

Common indentations (normal variants)

Cricopharyngeus muscle — posterior indentation at C6
Post-cricoid venous plexus — anterior indentation at C6
Aberrant right subclavian artery — posterior indentation at T2
Aortic knuckle — left-sided indentation at T4
Left main bronchus — oval impression, below the aortic knuckle
Left atrium — anterior impression on the lower third of the oesophagus
(pathological finding)

Oesophageal rings

'A' ring — marks the site of the lower oesophageal sphincter narrowing at the
upper end of the phrenic ampulla

'B' ring — oesophagogastric junction and is normally only seen with a hiatus hernia
(Schatzki/Templeton ring)

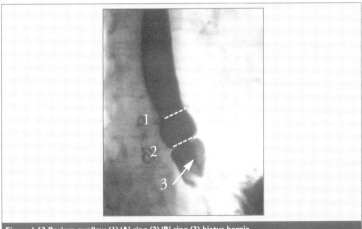

Figure 1.63 Barium swallow (1) 'A' ring (2) 'B' ring (3) hiatus hernia

'C' ring — proportion of the oesophagus seen within the abdominal cavity and is
normally 1-3 cm long

'Z' line — demarcates the junction of gastric and oesophageal mucosa

Oesophageal motility

Consists of three types of peristaltic waves:
1. primary wave — normal stripping wave associated with deglutition
2. secondary wave — normal stripping wave associated with oesophageal distension due to the presence of a food bolus
3. tertiary wave — non-peristaltic wave with a segmental appearance, possibly associated with a degree of dysmotility

Stomach

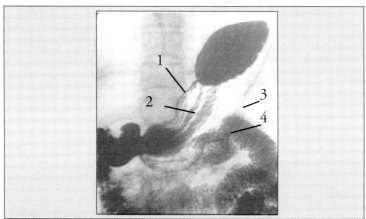

Figure 1.64 Barium meal (1) lesser curvature (2) magenstrasse (3) greater curvature (4) duodenojejunal flexure

Peritoneal attachments

Lesser omentum
From the inferior surface of the liver to the lesser curve of the stomach

Greater omentum
Free double layer of peritoneum extending from the greater curve of the stomach
Forms the gastrosplenic ligaments containing the short gastric and left gastroepiploic vessels

Radiological appearance (with double-contrast studies)

Area gastricae
Fine nodular elevation of the gastric mucosa (2-3 mm)
Found predominantly in the antrum

Rugae
Normal folds of mucosa (3-5 mm) following the curvature of the stomach

Magenstrasse
Folds parallelling the lesser curvature
Formed by the fibres of the oblique muscle layer
Most pronounced on erect views

Anterior	Anterior abdominal wall, diaphragm, left lobe of liver
Posterior	Diaphragm, lesser sac, spleen, left kidney, adrenal gland pancreas, transverse mesocolon, colon
Superior	Lesser omentum, right and left gastric vessels
Inferior	Greater omentum, right and left gastroepiploic vessels

Table 1.61 Relations of the stomach

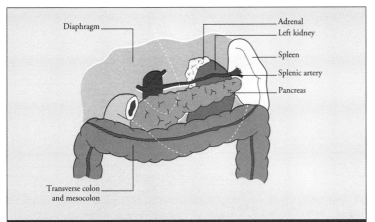

Figure 1.65 The posterior relations of the stomach
Reprinted from Clinical Anatomy, Ellis, pt. 2, The Abdomen and Pelvis, page 76: figure 52, 1997, by permission of Blackwell Science Ltd.

Vascular supply

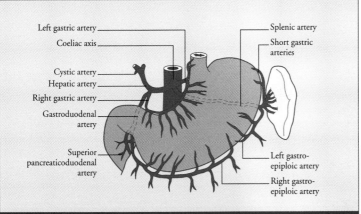

Figure 1.66 The arterial supply of the stomach
Reprinted from Clinical Anatomy, Ellis, pt. 2, The Abdomen and Pelvis, page 76: figure 53, 1997, by permission of Blackwell Science Ltd.

Pyloric anatomy (ultrasound appearances)

Mucosa of the pyloric canal is normal echogenic, the muscle echo-poor
Normal pyloric thickness is up to 4 mm, normal length is 18 mm
If the length is >18 mm and with the correct clinical symptoms, a diagnosis of
pyloric stenosis can be made

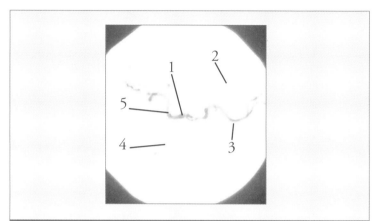

**Figure 1.67 Coeliac axis (1) common hepatic artery (2) left gastric artery (3) splenic artery
(4) gastroduodenal artery (5) hepatic artery proper**

Duodenum

Four parts, measuring 5 cm, 7.5 cm, 10 cm and 2.5 cm, respectively
Begins at L1, descends as far as L3 before rising to L2 at the duodenojejunal (DJ)
flexure
Proximal 2 cm of the first part and the distal 2 cm of the fourth part are
intraperitoneal, the remainder of the duodenum is retroperitoneal

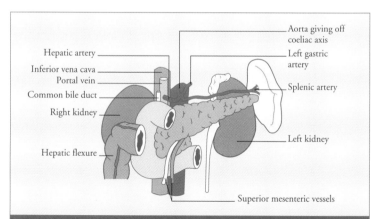

Figure 1.68 The relations of the duodenum
*Reprinted from Clinical Anatomy, Ellis, pt. 2, The Abdomen and Pelvis, page 80: figure 57, 1997, by permission of
Blackwell Science Ltd.*

First part	
Anterior	Liver, gallbladder
Posterior	Lesser sac, head of pancreas, portal vein, common bile duct, gastroduodenal artery
Superior	Portal vein, hepatic artery (all contained in the free edge of the lesser omentum), caudate lobe
Second part	
Anterior	Transverse colon, mesocolon, jejunum, liver
Posterior	Right kidney, right adrenal gland, IVC, head of pancreas, common bile duct, pancreaticoduodenal vessels
Third part	
Anterior	Small bowel, small-bowel mesentery, superior mesenteric vessels
Posterior	Aorta, IVC, inferior mesenteric artery, right ureter, right gonadal vessels
Fourth part	
Anterior	Small bowel, small-bowel mesentery
Posterior	Left kidney, left ureter, left renal and gonadal vessels
Superior	Body of pancreas

Table 1.62 Relations of the duodenum

Vascular anatomy
Pancreaticoduodenal vessels (coeliac trunk, superior mesenteric artery)

Small bowel
Extends from the DJ flexure to the ileocaecal junction
6 m in length
Root of the mesentery runs from the left of L2 to the right sacroiliac joint
(15 cm long)

Radiological appearances (contrast studies)

Jejunum
Proximal small bowel (40% of total small bowel)
Single vascular arcade
3.0-3.5 cm in diameter
Prominent valvulae coniventes (2-3 mm circular folds)

Ileum
Distal small bowel (60% of total small bowel)
Multiple vascular arcades
2.0-2.5 cm in diameter
Numerous Peyer's patches (lymphoid nodules)

Vascular supply

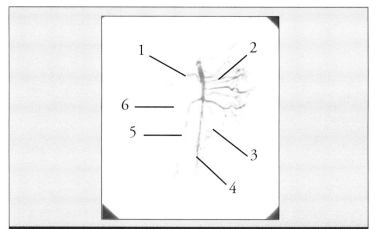

Figure 1.69 Superior mesenteric artery angiogram (1) middle colic artey (2) jejunal branches (3) ileal branches (4) continuation of the superior mesenteric artery (5) ileocolic artery (6) right colic artery

Appendix
Found at the convergence of the taeniae coli, a few centimetres below the ileocaecal valve on the posteromedial wall of the caecum
Exhibits no peristalsis
Visualized in the supine position during a barium enema

Meckel's diverticulum
Persistent remnant of the vitello-intestinal duct
Located on the anti-mesenteric border
5 cm long
Found 0.6 m from the ileocaecal valve
Affects 2% of the population

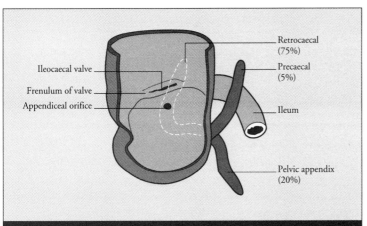

Ileocaecal valve
Frenulum of valve
Appendiceal orifice
Retrocaecal (75%)
Precaecal (5%)
Ileum
Pelvic appendix (20%)

Figure 1.610 Internal view of the caecum, showing the ileocaecal valve and the position of the appendix
Reprinted from Anatomy for Diagnostic Imaging, Ryan & McNichols, chapter 5, page 161: figure 5.16, 1994, by permission of WB Saunders Company.

Large intestine
Total length of approximately 1.6 m
Maximum normal diameter of the transverse colon is 5.5 cm and of the caecum is 9 cm
Taeniae coli consists of three flattened bands of longitudinal muscle that extend around the large bowel (except for the appendix and rectum, where there is a complete muscular cover)
Ascending and descending colon are retroperitoneal
Transverse and sigmoid colon have mesenteries

	Caecum	Ascending colon	Transverse colon	Descending colon
Anterior	Small bowel	Small bowel	Stomach Liver Gall bladder Spleen	Small bowel
Posterior	Gonadal vessels	Right kidney	Small bowel Second part of duodenum Head of pancreas	Diaphragm Left kidney

Table 1.63 Relations of the colon

Vascular anatomy

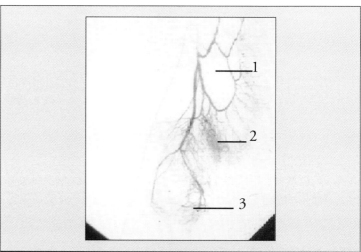

Figure 1.611 Inferior mesenteric artery angiogram (1) left colic artery (2) sigmoid artery (3) superior rectal artery

Liver

Anatomical division
Along the line of the falciform ligament and ligamentum teres

Morphological division
Along the line of the gall-bladder fossa and IVC (principal plane)

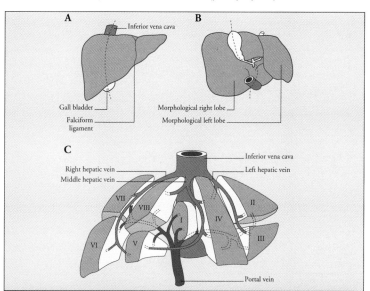

Figure 1.612 The morphological right and left lobes of the liver shown separated by the dotted line (A) anterior and (B) ventral aspect; note that the quadrate lobe is morphologically a part of the left lobe while the caudate lobe belongs to both the right and left lobes (C) the further segmental divisions of the liver
Reprinted from Clinical Anatomy, Ellis, pt. 2, The Abdomen and Pelvis, page 103: figure 72, 1997, by permission of Blackwell Science Ltd.

Segmental anatomy (Couinard classification)
Based on the hepatic veins and portal venous system
Each segment has a triad containing a portal vein, hepatic artery and bile duct
Hepatic veins do not follow this pattern but are segmental in their distribution

Riedel's lobe (normal variant)
Extended right lobe
Associated with an atrophic left lobe
More common in women

Peritoneal covering of the liver
Almost complete except for a bare area where the liver is in direct contact with the diaphragm
Four ligamentous attachments: right and left triangular ligaments, falciform ligament, coronary ligament

Vascular anatomy

Arterial supply

Hepatic artery

Forms 25% of the total blood supply of the liver

Arises from the coeliac trunk in 88% of the population (64% dorsal, 24% ventral to the common bile duct)

12% arise as an aberrant vessel from the superior mesenteric artery (SMA)

SMA

Supplies:

1. the entire liver in 2.5% of the population
2. part of the liver in 6% of the population
3. the right lobe in 10% of the population

Venous drainage

Hepatic veins

Central veins unite to form the right, middle and left hepatic veins, which converge on the bare area of the liver

Drain into the IVC

Portal vein

Responsible for 75% of the blood supply of the liver

Left portal vein runs anteriorly

Carries blood from the gastrointestinal tract to the liver

Portosystemic anastomoses are of pathological importance

Caudate lobe drains directly into the IVC

Biliary system

Conveys bile from the liver to the duodenum

Right and left hepatic ducts unite to form the common hepatic duct at the porta-hepatis (anterior to the hepatic artery and portal vein respectively)

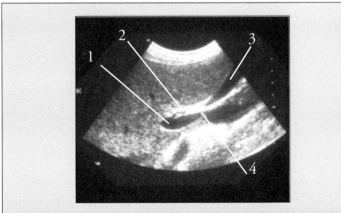

Figure 1.613 Longitudinal abdominal ultrasound (1) portal vein (2) hepatic artery (3) gall bladder (4) common bile duct (5) liver

Gall bladder

Concentrates and stores the bile

Covered by peritoneum except where it is attached to the visceral surface of the liver

Volume: 30-50 ml

Daily bile production: 500-1000 ml

Has a fundus, body and neck

Within the neck is the spiral valve of Heister (fold of mucosa with no smooth muscle)

The cystic duct is approximately 3 cm long with a normal diameter of 5-7 mm (up to 1 cm post-cholecystectomy)

The cystic duct unites with the common hepatic duct to form the common bile duct

The common bile duct descends in the free edge of the lesser omentum in direct relation to the head of the pancreas

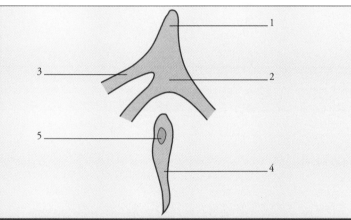

Figure 1.614 Duodenal ampullary folds (1) proximal longitudinal fold (2) hooding fold (3) oblique fold (4) distal longitudinal fold (5) ampulla

Pancreas

Mixed endocrine and exocrine gland

Retroperitoneal organ lying on the posterior abdominal wall

Positioned in the loop formed by the duodenum

Consists of a head, neck, body and tail

Directed obliquely upwards and to the left

Tail lies within the lienorenal ligament

Embryology

Ventral bud (foregut) produces the uncinate process and main pancreatic duct

Dorsal bud (midgut) forms the head, body and tail of the pancreas, as well as the accessory pancreatic duct

Variations include annular pancreas, pancreas divisum and accessory nodules

Radiological appearances

Identifiable by the splenic artery running along its upper border and the splenic vein posteriorly

Ultrasound shows increased echogenicity with age as the normal pancreas is replaced by fat

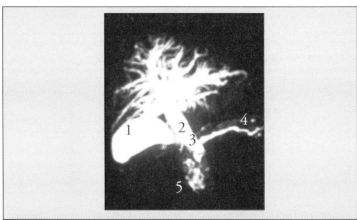

Figure 1.615 MRCP (pathological intra- and extrahepatic duct dilatation) (1) gall bladder (2) common hepatic duct (3) common bile duct (4) pancreatic duct (5) duodenum

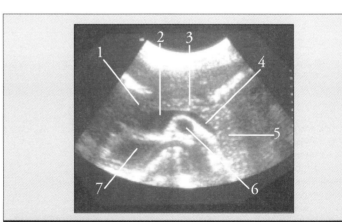

Figure 1.616 Transverse abdominal ultrasound (1) pancreatic head (2) portal vein confluence (3) pancreatic body (4) splenic vein (5) pancreatic tail (6) superior mesenteric artery (7) inferior vena cava

Vascular anatomy
Arterial supply
Pancreaticoduodenal arteries from the coeliac axis and superior mesenteric artery
Transverse pancreatic artery, great pancreatic artery, dorsal pancreatic artery and
pancreatic branches of the splenic artery

Venous drainage
Pancreaticoduodenal veins and splenic vein drain into the portal vein

	Head	Uncinate process	Neck	Body	Tail
Anterior	First part of duodenum Lesser sac Transverse colon Small bowel	Superior mesenteric vessels	Stomach Lesser sac Gastroduodenal artery Pancreatico-duodenal vessels	Stomach Lesser sac Small bowel Transverse colon	
Posterior	IVC Common bile duct Right renal vein	Left renal vessels	Portal vein confluence Superior mesenteric vessels	Aorta Splenic vein Inferior mesenteric vein Left kidney Left adrenal gland	
Inferior	Third part of duodenum	Third part of duodenum		DJ flexure	
Right/left	Second part of duodenum				Hilum of the spleen

Table 1.64 Relations of the pancreas

Spleen
Lymphoid and haemopoietic organ
Lies in the left hypochondrium
Related to the 9th, 10th and 11th ribs
Dimensions: 12 x 7 x 7 cm with the long axis along the 10th rib
Almost entirely covered by peritoneum, with attachments via the gastrosplenic
ligament anteriorly (short gastric and gastroepiploic vessels) and lienorenal
ligament posteriorly (splenic vessels and tail of pancreas)

Splenunculi (pancreatic tail, small-bowel mesentery, greater omentum) seen in 10%
of the population

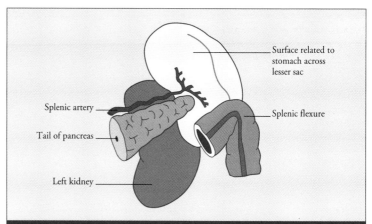

Figure 1.617 The spleen and its immediate relations
Reprinted from Clinical Anatomy, Ellis, pt. 2, The Abdomen and Pelvis, page 111: figure 79, 1997, by permission of Blackwell Science Ltd.

Vascular anatomy
Arterial supply
Splenic artery — arises from the coeliac axis

Venous drainage
Splenic vein forms the portal vein with the superior mesenteric vein behind the neck of the pancreas

Anterior	Stomach
Posterior	Left kidney, left adrenal gland
Inferior	Splenic flexure
Medial	Tail of the pancreas

Table 1.65 Relations of the spleen

Kidneys

Retroperitoneal organs in the paravertebral gutters
Lie obliquely
Long axis is directed upwards, medially and backward
Size in adults: 3.5 lumbar vertebrae and discs (children, 4.5)
Ultrasound range: 9-12 cm
IVU range: 12-16 cm
A difference of ≤1.5 cm between the left and right kidney is normal
Left kidney is usually larger than the right

Hilar

Right hilum is at the level of L2
Left hilum is at the level of the L1/L2 disc

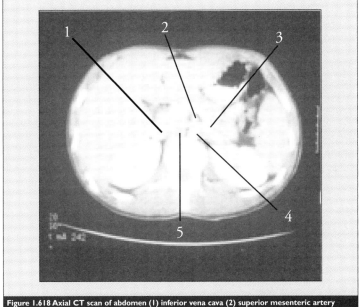

Figure 1.618 Axial CT scan of abdomen (1) inferior vena cava (2) superior mesenteric artery (3) left renal vein (4) aorta (5) right crus

Hilar structures (anterior→posterior)

Renal vein
Renal artery
Ureter
(Renal artery)

Fascial spaces

Kidneys, adrenals and peri-renal fat pads are enclosed within the renal fascia
Gerota's fascia — anterior lamella of the renal fascia
Fascia of Zuckerkandl — posterior lamella of the renal fascia
Limit the spread of renal-associated infection

Embryological variants

Persistent foetal lobulation — surface notches between the calyces
Horseshoe kidney — detected by abnormal configuration of pelvicocalyceal (PC) systems and the presence of preaortic renal tissue
Ectopic pelvic kidney
Crossed fused ectopia — the right kidney is correctly positioned and its lower pole is fused with the upper pole of the left kidney, which is mutated across the midline
Duplex system:
    1. partial/complete
    2. upper moiety obstructs; lower refluxes
Retrocaval ureter — the ureter is seen to be displaced medially

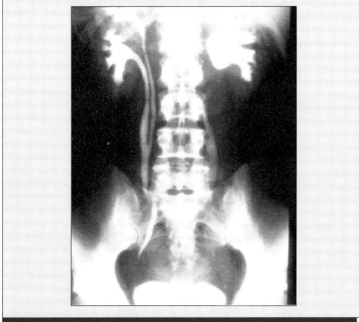

Figure 1.619 IVU: partial right duplex system

	Right kidney	Left kidney
Anterior	Liver Duodenum Colon Small bowel	Spleen Stomach Pancreas Colon Small bowel
Posterior	Diaphragm Posterior abdominal wall	Diaphragm Posterior abdominal wall
Medial	Renal vessels Ureter IVC	Left adrenal gland Renal vessels Ureter Aorta
Superior	Right adrenal gland	

Table 1.66 Relations of the kidneys

Vascular anatomy

Arterial supply

Renal arteries arises at the level of L1/L2

Right renal artery is posterior to the IVC (longitudinal ultrasound section)

Renal arteries divides into three branches — upper posterior, upper anterior and lower

Subdivided into five segmental branches

25% of the population have multiple renal arteries arising directly from the aorta

Venous drainage

Directly into the IVC

Left renal vein receives the left inferior phrenic, left adrenal and left gonadal veins

Left renal vein is an anterior relation to the aorta and posterior to the SMA

Ureters

Muscular tubes draining urine from the kidneys to the bladder
Retroperitoneal structures both in the abdomen and pelvis
Approximately 25 cm long

Abdominal portion		
	Left	**Right**
Anterior	Second part of the duodenum Root of the small-bowel mesentery Right colic vessels Ileocolic vessels Right gonadal vessels	Sigmoid mesocolon Colic vessels Left gonadal vessels
Pelvic portion		
	Right	**Left**
Anterosuperior	Vas deferens Broad ligament Uterine artery Ovary	Vas deferens Broad ligament Uterine artey Ovary
Posterior	Sacroiliac joint Common iliac vessels	Sacroiliac joint Common iliac vessels
Medial	Seminal vesicle Lateral fornix	Seminal vesicle Lateral fornix

Table 1.67 Relations of the ureters

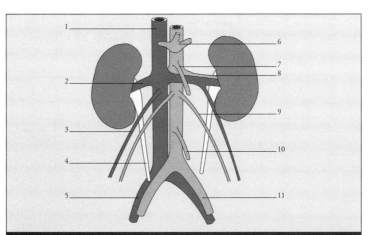

Figure 1.620 Posterior abdominal wall structures (1) inferior vena cava (2) right renal vein (3) right gonadal vein (4) right ureter (5) right common iliac vein (6) coeliac axis (7) superior mesenteric artery (8) left renal artery (9) left gonadal artery (10) inferior mesenteric artery (11) left common iliac artery

Vascular anatomy
Arterial supply
Aortic, renal and gonadal arteries
Internal iliac, vesical and uterine arteries

Venous drainage
Follows the arterial supply

Adrenal glands
Endocrine glands on the posterior abdominal wall
Dimensions: 4 × 3 × 1 cm
Although enclosed in renal fascia, the glands are separated from the kidneys by fat
Right gland is triangular, in direct relation with the superior pole of the right kidney
Left gland is crescentic, in direct relation with the medial border of the left kidney
In transverse section, both glands are 'Y' shaped, the posteromedial limb of which is the largest

Development
At birth, the adrenal glands are one-third the size of the kidney
In adulthood, they are 1/30th the size of the kidney

Vascular anatomy
Arterial supply
Inferior phrenic artery
Aorta
Renal artery

Venous drainage
Right adrenal vein drains directly into the IVC
Left adrenal vein drains via the left renal vein

Abdominal aorta
Pierces the diaphragm at the level of T12
Descends to the left of the midline to the level of L4, where it divides into the common iliac arteries
Three unpaired anterior branches — coeliac trunk, superior and inferior mesenteric arteries
Three paired visceral lateral branches — suprarenal, renal and gonadal
Five paired parietal branches — inferior phrenic and four lumbar arteries
Terminal branches — median sacral artery and common iliac arteries

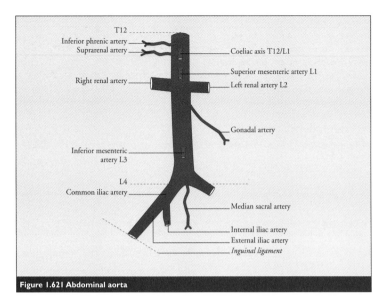

Figure 1.621 Abdominal aorta

IVC

Formed at the level of L5 by the union of the common iliac veins

Ascends to the right of the midline

Crossed by the right common iliac artery

Pierces the diaphragm at the level of T8

No valves except for the rudimentary semilunar valve at the entrance of the right atrium

Connected to the azygos venous system via the lumbar veins

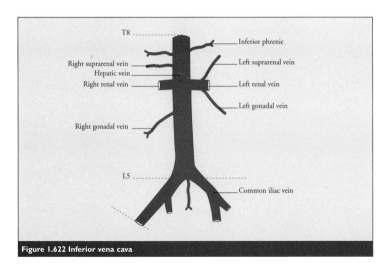

Figure 1.622 Inferior vena cava

Portal vein

Drains venous blood from the gastrointestinal tract, pancreas and spleen
Formed at the confluence of the superior mesenteric vein and splenic vein behind
the neck of the pancreas (L1/L2 disc)
Runs in the free edge of the lesser momentum to enter the liver at the porta
hepatis

Cisterna chyli

Proximal dilated thoracic duct
Length: 6 cm
Anterior to L1, L2
Drains via the thoracic duct (38-45 cm long)

1.7 The Pelvis

Bony anatomy

Two innominate bones (each made up of ilium, ischium and pubis), sacrum and coccyx
Pubic symphysis is a secondary cartilaginous joint with a normal width of <7 mm
Sacroiliac joints are planar synovial joints; they are atypical in that they have
fibrocartilage rather than hyaline cartilage on the joint surface

Sex differences

Male
Heart-shaped outline
Infrapubic angle of approximately 90°

Female
Oval outline
Infrapubic angle >120°

Pelvic floor

Formed by levator ani and the coccygeus complex
Perineal body — fibromuscular node, posterior to the urethra in the male and to
the urethra and vagina in the female
Anococcygeal body — fibromuscular node between the anus and the coccyx

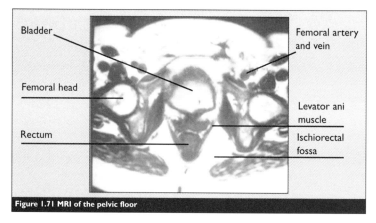

Bladder
Femoral artery and vein
Femoral head
Levator ani muscle
Rectum
Ischiorectal fossa

Figure 1.71 MRI of the pelvic floor

Ischiorectal fossa (ischioanal fossa)

Wedge-shaped space filled with fat
Situated:
    1. below and lateral to levator ani and the anal canal
    2. medial to the inner wall of the pelvis and obturator internus
Anteriorly limited by the perineal body
Free communication between both sides
Contents:
    1. ischiorectal fat pad
    2. pudendal canal (of Alcock), pudendal nerve and internal pudendal vessels
    3. minor vessels and nerves

Sigmoid colon and rectum

Sigmoid colon

Approximately 40 cm long
Attached to the posterior and left lateral pelvic wall by a mesentery,
the apex of which is a direct relation to the left sacroiliac joint

Relations

Left ureter
Bifurcation of the left common iliac artery
Superior rectal vessels

Rectum

Approximately 12 cm long
Extends from S3 to C4
Rectosigmoid junction is at the level of S3

Peritoneal covering

Upper third — peritoneum anteriorly and laterally
Middle third — peritoneum anteriorly
Lower third — entirely retroperitoneal

Mucosal pattern

Longitudinal folds of mucosa form the columns of Morgagni (3 mm wide)
Horizontal folds form the valves of Houston (5 mm wide)

Common iliac arteries

Commence at the bifurcation of the aorta (L4)
Divide into the internal and external iliac arteries in front of the sacroiliac joints
Right common iliac artery is longer than the left common iliac artery and is an
anterior relation of the inferior vena cava (IVC)

External iliac artery

Commences at the level of the sacroiliac joints
Runs along the pelvic brim on the medial border of psoas
Passes beneath the inguinal ligament (halfway between the anterior superior iliac
spine and pubic symphysis: midinguinal point) to enter the femoral sheath

Branches

Occur above the inguinal ligament:
  1. inferior epigastric artery
  2. deep circumflex iliac artery

Relations

Crossed anteriorly by the ureter
Gonadal vessels
External iliac vein commences posteriorly but comes to lie medial to the artery

Internal iliac artery

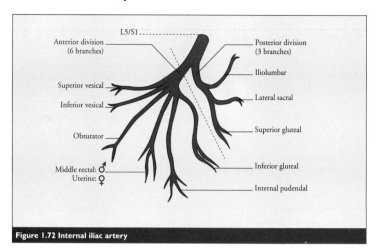

Figure 1.72 Internal iliac artery

Forms an anterior and posterior division
Anterior division supplies the pelvic viscera, perineum and hip joint
Posterior division supplies the spinal cord, vertebral column and gluteal
muscles

Anterior (female)	Ureter (fallopian tube and ovary)
Posterior	Internal iliac vein, lumbosacral trunk and sacroiliac joint
Lateral	External iliac artery and vein, obturator nerve
Medial	Parietal peritoneum, small bowel

Table 1.71 Relations of the internal iliac artery

Iliac veins
Correspond to the arteries and their branches
Unite to form the IVC at the level of L5 behind the right common iliac artery

Pelvic ureters

Enter the pelvis anterior to psoas and the bifurcation of the iliac vessels
Run on the lateral wall of the pelvis
At the level of the ischial spine, turn medially

Male relations

The ureter is above the seminal vesicles
Crossed by the vas deferens anteriorly

Female relations

The ureter is above the lateral fornix of the vagina
Lateral to the cervix
Inferior to the uterine vessels in the broad ligament
Enters the posterolateral aspect of the bladder with an oblique intramural passage

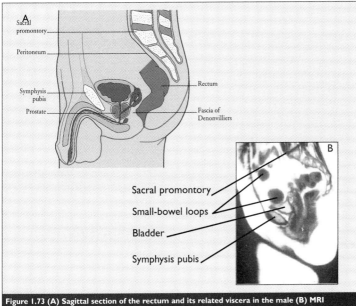

Figure 1.73 (A) Sagittal section of the rectum and its related viscera in the male (B) MRI

Bladder

Form and size is the same in both sexes
Intra-abdominal organ in children
Three-sided pyramid with a capacity of approximately 300 ml
The trigone is a triangular area at the base of the bladder between the internal urethral orifice and the two ureteral orifices
Ureteric orifices are connected by a transverse ridge called the interureteric bar
Peritoneal reflections differ between males and females:

1. males — the superior portion is covered by peritoneum
2. females — only the anterior portion is covered by peritoneum, the remainder lies in direct relation with the uterus

	Male	Female
Superior	Sigmoid colon Small bowel	Uterus Sigmoid colon Small bowel
Inferior	Prostate gland	Levator ani Pubic bones
Posterior	Seminal vesicles Vas deferens Rectum	Vagina Cervix

Table 1.72 Relations of the bladder

Male pelvis
Prostate gland

Cone-shaped with inner glandular and outer fibrous structure
Consists of anterior, posterior, lateral and median lobes
Traversed vertically by the urethra
Ejaculatory ducts and prostatic ducts open onto the posterior prostatic urethra at the level of the verumontanum

Superior	Bladder
Posterior	Rectum
Inferolateral	Levator ani and pubic bones

Table 1.73 Relations of the prostate gland

Male urethra

Prostatic urethra
3 cm long
Widest part of the urethra

Membranous urethra
2 cm long
Narrowest portion of the urethra
Traverses the urogenital diaphragm

Bulbous urethra
Surrounded by the corpus spongiosum

Penile urethra
16 cm long
Lies within the corpus spongiosum of the penis
Narrow except at the area of the navicular fossa

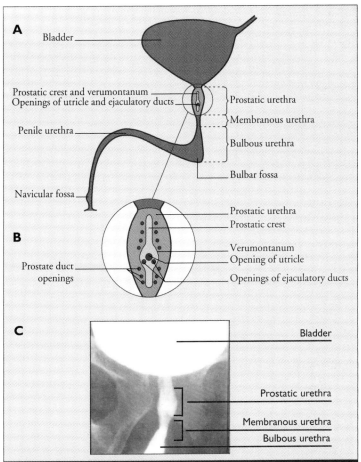

Figure 1.75 Male bladder and urethra (A) sagittal section (B) prostatic urethra showing ducts (C) urethrogram

(A,B)Reprinted from Anatomy for Diagnostic Imaging, Ryan & McNichols, chapter 6, page 219: figure 6.12, 1994, by permission of WB Saunders Company.

Testes
Approximately 4 x 2.5 x 3 cm
Surrounded by the visceral layer of the tunica vaginalis except posterolaterally, where it is in direct contact with the epididymis
Epididymis is a coiled tube with its head at the superior pole and its tail at the inferior pole of the testis

Spermatic cord
Three fascial layers (external spermatic, cremasteric, internal spermatic)
Three arteries (testicular, cremasteric, vas deferens)
Three other structures (pampiniform plexus, vas deferens, lymph vessels — para-aortic nodes)

Female pelvis
Uterus
Approximately 8 × 5 × 3 cm
Comprised of a fundus, body and cervix
Receives the uterine tubes
Cervix opens into the vault of the vagina
Covered by peritoneum except on the inferior surface, where it is in direct contact with the bladder
Anterior reflection forms the uterovesical pouch and the posterior reflection forms the rectouterine pouch (of Douglas)

Anterior	Bladder
Posterior	Rectouterine pouch, rectum, posterior fornix
Superior	Sigmoid colon, small bowel
Inferior	Vagina
Lateral	Uterine tubes, ovaries, broad ligaments

Table 1.74 Relations of the uterus

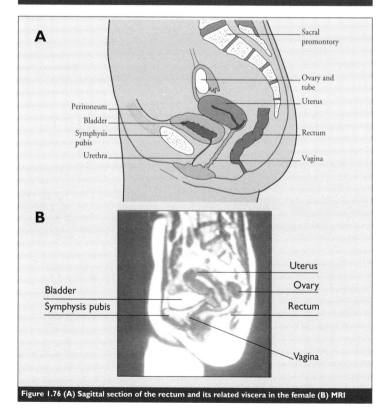

Figure 1.76 (A) Sagittal section of the rectum and its related viscera in the female (B) MRI

Ligaments

Broad ligament

Double fold of the peritoneum but not a true ligament

Extends from the side wall of the uterus to the lateral wall of the pelvis

Upper border is free

Contains the uterine tube and vessels, and the ovarian and round ligaments

Round ligament

Fibromuscular band

Extends from the junction of the uterus to the deep inguinal ring

Continuous with the ligament of the ovary

Continues through the inguinal canal and is attached to the labium majus of the vulva

Ovarian ligament

Continuous with the round ligament

Attached to the corresponding ovary

Carries the ovarian vessels and lymphatics

Others

Lateral, uterosacral ligaments

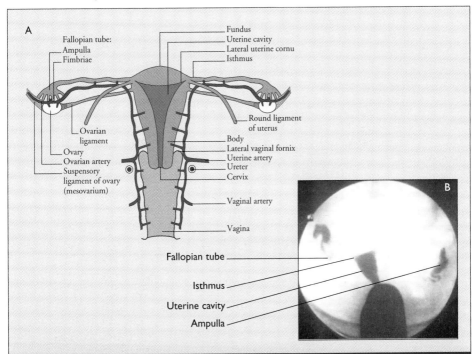

Figure 1.77 (A) Uterus and fallopian tubes: coronal section showing blood supply and ureter relative to uterine artery, cervix and vagina (B) Hysterosalpingogram

(A) Reprinted from Anatomy for Diagnostic Imaging, Ryan & McNichols, chapter 6, page 226: figure 6.19, 1994, by permission of WB Saunders Company.

Ovaries

Size: 2 × 3 × 4 cm

Situated in the posterior aspect of the broad ligament

Attached to the infundibulum of the uterine tube

Ultrasound appearances:
1. pre-menarche: smooth, homogeneous
2. childbearing age: multiple cysts/follicles
3. post-menopause: small, atrophic, with no evidence of follicular development

Uterine tube

Approximately 10 cm long

Consists of four segments
1. uterine segment
2. isthmus (narrow)
3. ampulla
4. infundibulum

Lies in the superior border of the broad ligament

Female urethra

4 cm long

Embedded in the vaginal wall

No internal urethral sphincter

1.8 The Upper Limb

Clavicle
Ossifies in membrane with no medullary cavity
First bone to ossify
Secondary ossification centre appears at the sternal end
0.6% of the population have a rhomboid fossa medially for attachment to the costoclavicular ligament
Conoid tubercle gives attachment laterally to the coracoclavicular ligament

Scapula
Extends inferiorly to the 7th interspace
Seven secondary ossification centres

Shoulder

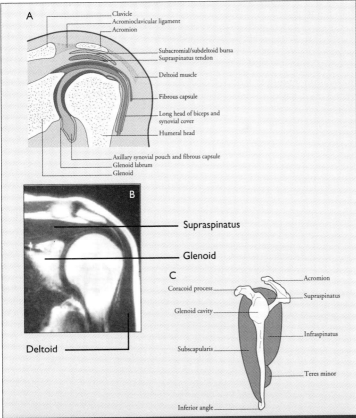

Figure 1.81 **(A) Coronal section through the shoulder joint as seen on coronal MRI scan (B) MRI scan (C) rotator cuff**
(A) Reprinted from Anatomy for Diagnostic Imaging, Ryan & McNichols, chapter 7, page 244: figure 7.9, 1994, by permission of WB Saunders Company.
(C) Reprinted from Grant's Atlas of Anatomy, 9th Edition, Agur, chapter 6, page 394: figure 6.51, 1991, by permission of Williams and Wilkins.

Synovial ball-and-socket joint involving the humeral head and glenoid cavity
Humeral head has a greater tuberosity (posterolateral) and a lesser tuberosity
They are separated by the intertubercular groove, through which passes the long
head of the biceps (intrasynovial)

Greater tuberosity has attachments for supraspinatus, infraspinatus and teres
minor (superior to inferior)
Lesser tuberosity gives attachment to subscapularis
These four muscles form the rotator cuff
Glenoid cavity is deepened by the ring of fibrocartilage called the glenoid labrum
The long heads of the biceps and triceps are attached to the superior and
inferior tubercle of the cavity
The capsule of the shoulder joint is attached proximally to the glenoid labrum
and distally to the humeral head and neck — it is lax inferiorly
The bursae of the shoulder joint are the subacromial and subscapular, of
which the subscapular normally communicates with the joint space

Radiological development of the shoulder

The greater and lesser tuberosities and humeral head ossify in years 1, 2 and 5,
respectively
The coracoid process has two epiphyses

Radiography of the shoulder

10% of the population show failure of fusion of the acromion (os acromiale)
The normal acromiohumeral distance is $\geq$7 mm — a reduction in this distance is
seen with rotator-cuff tears

Elbow

Expansion of the distal humerus to form lateral and medial epicondyles
Capitellum and trochlea articulate with the radius and ulna, respectively
Elbow joint consists of only one cavity
It has an anterior and posterior fat pad — elevation of the posterior pad is always
pathological

Ossification centre	Age of appearance (years)
Capitellum	1
Radial head	3
Internal epicondyle	5
Trochlea	9-11
Olecranon	9-11
Lateral epicondyle	9-11

Table 1.81 Radiological development of the elbow

Epiphyses fuse together at puberty and with the shaft at 17 years

Radiography of the elbow

Normal carrying angle: males 168°, females 170°

In the lateral view, at least one-third of the capitellum should be anterior to the long axis of the humerus (posterior displacement occurs with supracondylar fractures)

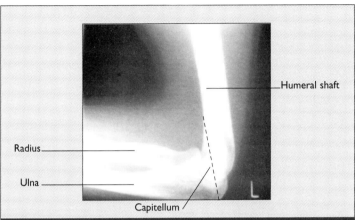

Radius

Ulna

Capitellum

Humeral shaft

L

Figure 1.82 Lateral radiograph of elbow

Wrist and hand

In the neutral position, the radius articulates with the scaphoid and lunate

The ulna articulates with the radius and the triangular fibrocartilaginous complex (TFCC)

The triquetral is unsupported

The normal carpal angle is 124°-139°

The wrist and hand have three joints: the distal radioulnar, the radiocarpal and the midcarpal joints — they do not normally communicate

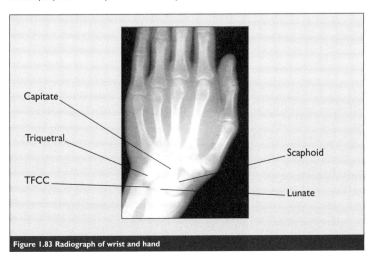

Capitate

Triquetral

TFCC

Scaphoid

Lunate

Figure 1.83 Radiograph of wrist and hand

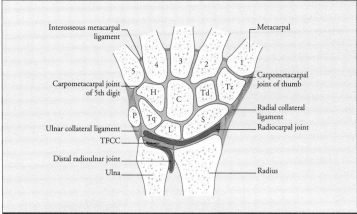

Fig 1.84 Bones and ligaments of the wrist
Reprinted from Grant's Atlas of Anatomy, 9th Edition, Agur, chapter 6, page 448: figure 6.138, 1991, by permission of Williams and Wilkins.

Carpal tunnel

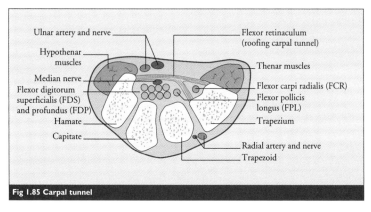

Fig 1.85 Carpal tunnel

The flexor retinaculum extends from the pisiform and hook of the hamate medially, to the scaphoid tubercle and the trapezium laterally

The FDS, FDP, FPL and median nerve pass through the carpal tunnel

The flexor carpi ulnaris, FCR, ulnar and radial neurovascular bundles are found outside the carpal tunnel

Radiological development of the carpal bones
Carpal bones ossify in sequence, beginning with the capitate

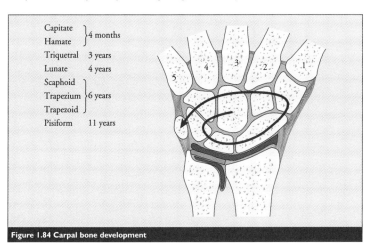

Capitate	} 4 months
Hamate	
Triquetral	3 years
Lunate	4 years
Scaphoid	} 6 years
Trapezium	
Trapezoid	
Pisiform	11 years

Figure 1.84 Carpal bone development

Arterial supply of the upper limb

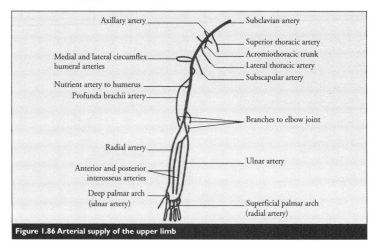

Figure 1.86 Arterial supply of the upper limb

Venous drainage of the upper limb

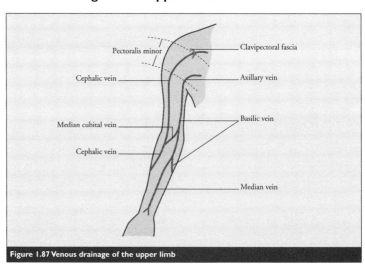

Figure 1.87 Venous drainage of the upper limb

1.9 The Lower Limb

Femur
Hemispherical head
Fovea capitus centrally positioned gives attachment to the ligamentum teres
Femoral neck forms an angle of inclination and anteversion in relation to the shaft:
　1. at birth — 160° and 50°, respectively
　2. in adult life — 127° and 8°, respectively

The distance between the femur and the acetabulum may be up to 11 mm in childhood, reducing to 4-7 mm in adults

Radiological development of the upper femur
Femoral head appears at the age of 1 year
Greater trochanter appears at 5 years
Lesser trochanter appears at 10 years
All fuse at 18 years of age

Hip
Ball-and-socket joint involving the head of the femur and acetabulum (formed by the ilium, ischium and pubis)
Joint capsule attached circumferentially — intertrochanteric line anteriorly; halfway along the femoral neck posteriorly
Strengthened by three ligaments — iliofemoral (strongest), pubofemoral and ischiofemoral

Radiography of the hip and pelvis
Shenton's line
Continuous line from the medial aspect of the femur and inferior aspect of the superior pubic ramus
Disrupted when pathology present

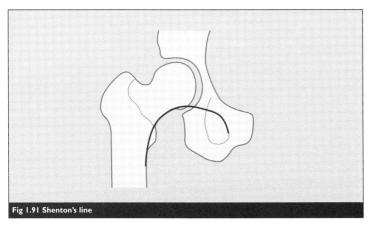

Fig 1.91 Shenton's line

Von Rosen's view
Anteroposterior (AP) with internal rotation and 45° abduction
Specifically used to look for congenital dislocation

Pelvimetry
AP inlet 11-13 cm
AP outlet 10-12 cm
Interspinous distance 9-11 cm

Femoral triangle
Surface marking of the femoral artery
The midinguinal point is halfway between the anterior superior iliac spine (ASIS) and the pubic symphysis

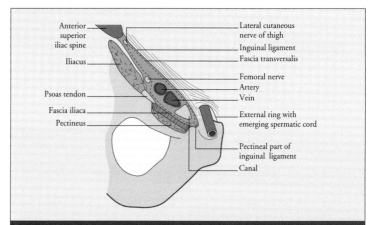

Figure 1.92 The femoral canal and its surrounds
Reprinted from Clinical Anatomy, Ellis, pt. 4, The Lower Limb, page 257: figure 175, 1997, by permission of Blackwell Science Ltd.

Knee
Synovial hinge joint involving femur, tibia and patella
Fibula articulates only with the posterolateral aspect of the tibia
Largest synovial cavity in the body

Fabella
Found in 25% of adults
Lies in the lateral head of gastrocnemius

Patella
Largest sesamoid bone, appearing at the age of 3 years
Three paired facets on the posterior surface
Bipartite patella seen in 10% of the population, with the superolateral aspect ossifying independently
Prone to lateral dislocation despite:
    1. anterior-placed lateral condyle of the femur
    2. horizontal insertion of vastus medialis

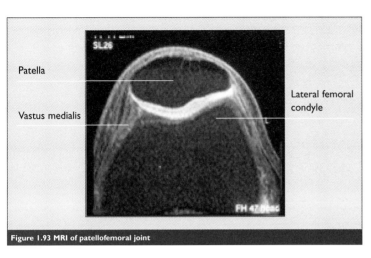

Patella

Lateral femoral condyle

Vastus medialis

Figure 1.93 MRI of patellofemoral joint

Radiological development of the knee
Lower femoral epiphysis observed at 37 weeks *in utero*
Upper tibial epiphysis present at birth
Patella visible at 3 years of age
Fusion of epiphysis occurs at approximately 18 years

Radiology of the knee
Joint space 3-8 mm
Patellofemoral distance 3 mm
Tunnel view:
    1. 90° posterior — intercondylar notch
    2. 110° anterior — intercondylar notch
Skyline view displays the articular surface of the patella

Knee ligaments
Medial collateral ligament
Broad band
Superficial and deep component
Attached to the capsule and medial meniscus

Lateral collateral ligament
Cord-like structure
Attached to the head of the fibula
Separate from the capsule and lateral meniscus

Anterior cruciate ligament (ACL)
Passes from the anterior intercondylar area to the medial surface of the lateral
femoral condyle and prevents posterior displacement of the femur on the tibia

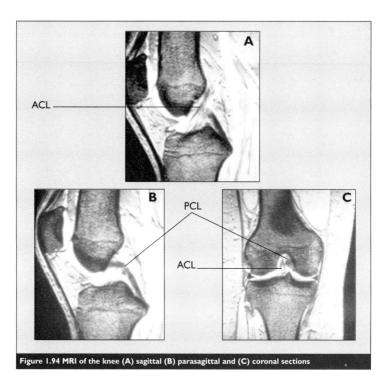

Figure 1.94 MRI of the knee (A) sagittal (B) parasagittal and (C) coronal sections

Posterior cruciate ligament (PCL)
Passes from the posterior intercondylar area to the lateral aspect of the medial femoral condyle and prevents anterior displacement of the femur on the tibia

Note: cruciates (and popliteus) are entirely intracapsular but extrasynovial

Coronary ligament
Provides attachment for both menisci to the tibia

Meniscofemoral ligaments
Anterior (Humphrey) and posterior (Risberg)
Straddle the posterior cruciate

Menisci

Avascular
Made of fibrocartilage
Attached to the tibial plateau by the coronary ligament
Wedge-shaped cross-section

Medial meniscus	Lateral meniscus
Larger	Smaller
Anterior thickness 6 mm	Uniform 10 mm thickness
Posterior thickness 14 mm	
Semicircular	Circular
Firm capsular attachment	Free from the capsule

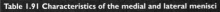

Table 1.91 Characteristics of the medial and lateral menisci

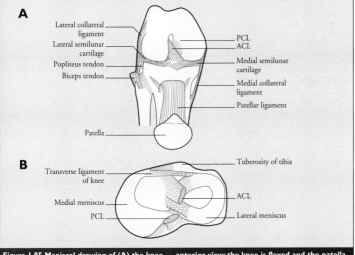

Figure 1.95 Meniscal drawing of (A) the knee — anterior view; the knee is flexed and the patella has been turned downwards (B) the right knee in transverse section

Synovial cavity

Divided into three, with all parts communicating freely

Seven bursae

Four communicating — suprapatellar, popliteus, gastrocnemius and semimembranosus
Three normally separate — prepatellar, infrapatellar (subcutaneous, deep)

Tibiofibular joint

Proximal joint is a plane synovial joint
Distal tibiofibular and talofibular joints are syndesmoses (fibrous)

Ankle joint and foot

Hinge joint of the tibia and fibula with the upper surface of the talus
Medial malleolus is shorter than the lateral malleolus
Capsule is attached to the articular margins — lax anteriorly

Ankle ligaments
Medial (deltoid) ligament
Superficial and deep component

Lateral ligament
Three parts — calcanofibular, anterior and posterior talofibular

Radiography of the ankle and foot
Lower limbs are varoid up to 2 years, then valgoid from 12 years onwards
Talotibial distance on a standard AP film is 3-5 mm
Epiphysis of the 5th metatarsal is parallel to the long axis (can mimic a fracture, normally perpendicular)

Bohler's angle
28°-40°
Normal talocalcaneal angle
Reduced in pathology

Heel-pad thickness
Males <23 mm
Females <21.5 mm

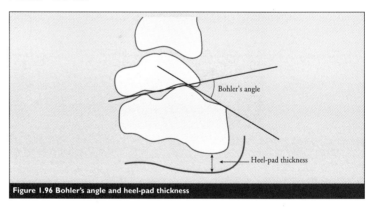

Bohler's angle

Heel-pad thickness

Figure 1.96 Bohler's angle and heel-pad thickness

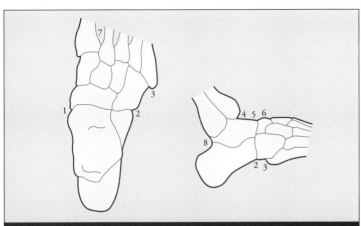

Figure 1.910 Accessory ossicles (1) os tibiale externum (2) os peroneum (3) os vesalianum (4) os talotibiale (5) os supratalare (6) os supranaviculare (7) os intermetatarseum (8) os trigonum

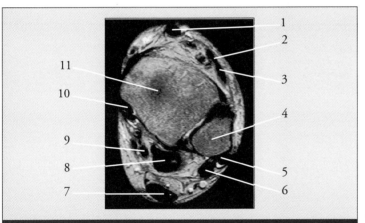

Figure 1.911 MRI through the lower leg — axial section (1) tibialis anterior (2) extensor hallucis longus (3) extensor digitorum longus (4) distal fibula (5) peroneus longus (6) peroneus brevis (7) tendocalcaneus (8) flexor hallucis longus (9) flexor digitorum longus (10) tibialis posterior (11) distal tibia

Arterial supply of the lower limb

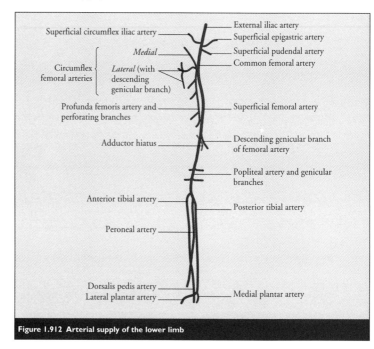

Figure 1.912 Arterial supply of the lower limb

Venous drainage of the lower limb

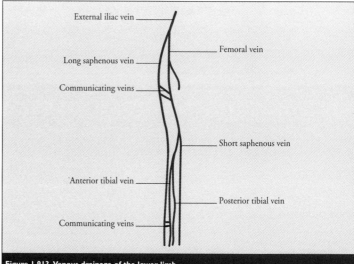

Figure 1.913 Venous drainage of the lower limb

Section Two
Basic Physics

2.1 The Atom

Mass number (A)
Number of protons and neutrons in the nucleus

Atomic number (Z)
Number of protons in the nucleus
Constant and determines the chemical characteristics of the element

Nucleus
Formed of protons and neutrons
Concerned with the production of radioactivity (γ-rays)

Electrons
Low-mass, negatively charged orbiting particles
Outer electron shells confer chemical and electrical properties to the atom
Inner electron shells are concerned with the production of X-rays
Number of electrons per shell = $2n^2$ (where n = shell number)

E (binding energy of the electron)
Energy expended in completely removing the electron from the atom
Proportional to the atomic number

Photon energy

$$E = hf$$

f = frequency of the radiation
h = Planck's constant (4.13×10^{-18} keV/s)

Electromagnetic radiation

Comprises both quantum (particulate) and waveform (transverse) energy
All types of electromagnetic radiation travel at the same speed in a vacuum
Consists of packets of energy called photons

Electromagnetic spectrum

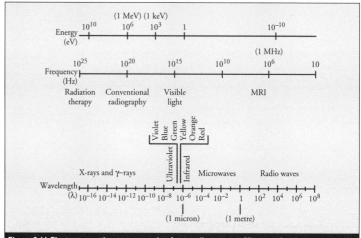

Figure 2.11 Electromagnetic spectra ranging from radio waves to X-rays and γ-rays

2.2 X-ray Tube Design

Construction of the X-ray tube

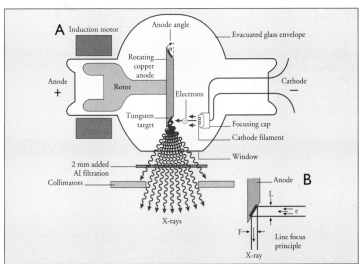

Figure 2.21 (A) Major components of an X-ray tube **(B)** The magnified view of the target illustrates the line focus principle — the focal spot size 'F' is smaller than the electron beam 'L' because of the anode angle

Filament
Made from tungsten (high Z)
Voltage 10 V; current 10 A
Undergoes thermionic emission by heating to 2200°C

Tube
Made of a glass envelope containing a vacuum
Accelerating voltage 30-150 kV; current 0.5-1000 mA
These are independent of each other
The tube current is proportional to the kV, temperature and the current of the filament

Target
Made of tungsten embedded in copper (to improve heat conduction)
+/- rhenium (to reduce pitting)
Electron stream penetrates a few microns into the target
This results in three processes:
   1. interaction with the outer electrons — produces heat
      (99% of electron-electron interactions)
   2. interaction with the inner electrons — produces X-rays
      (1% of electron-electron interactions)
   3. interaction with the nucleus — most X-rays are produced
      by bremsstrahlung process

Line focus principle

Focal spot is the area of the target bombarded by the electron stream
Anode angle (6°-20°) produces foreshortening of the apparent focal spot
Decreasing the angle produces a smaller apparent focal spot, so improving
anatomical detail (mammography)

Modality	Focal spot size (mm)
Macro mammography	0.1
Mammography	0.3
Macro radiography	0.3
Radiography	0.6-1.2
Fluoroscopy	0.6

Table 2.21 Typical focal spot size for specific modalities

Rotating anode speeds vary between 3,000 and 17,000 rpm

Heat dissipation

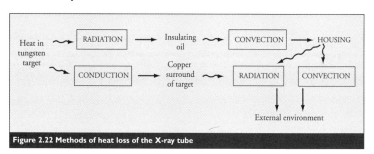

Figure 2.22 Methods of heat loss of the X-ray tube

Heat rating

$$\text{Heat rating (joules)} = kV \times mAs$$

This increases with effective focal spot, rotating anode and increased size of anode
disc
In fluoroscopy (continuous exposure), heat removal rate must be equivalent to
production rate

2.3 X-ray Production and Beam Properties

Characteristic radiation

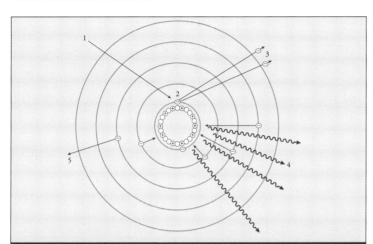

Figure 2.31 Characteristic radiation is produced when an incoming electron (1) interacts with an inner shell electron (2) and both are ejected (3); when one of the outer shell electrons moves to fill the inner shell vacancy, the excess energy is emitted as characteristic radiation (4); sometimes the excess energy is emitted as an Auger electron (5) rather than as characteristic radiation

Bremsstrahlung radiation (braking radiation)

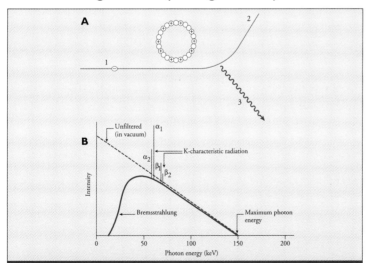

Figure 2.32 (A) Bremsstrahlung radiation is produced when an energetic electron (1) (with initial energy E_1) passes close to an atomic nucleus; the attractive force of the positively charged nucleus causes the electron to change direction and lose energy; the electron (2) now has a lower energy (E_2); the energy difference (E_1–E_2) is released as an X-ray photon (3): **(B)** The spectrum of bremsstrahlung and characteristic radiation

Bremsstrahlung radiation is responsible for 80% of X-rays in diagnostic imaging

kV	% total X-ray production
<70	0
70-150	10-28
>150	≈ 1

Table 2.31 Variation of characteristic radiation with kV

Properties of the X-ray beam

Quantity (intensity/air Kerma)
Proportional to Z, kV^2, mA and $1/d^2$ (where d = distance from target)
Increases with constant potential
Decreases with increasing filtration

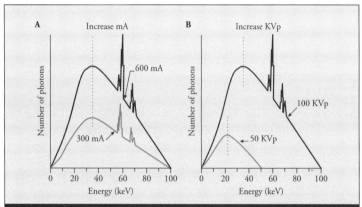

Figure 2.33 Effect of current and voltage on X-ray spectra: (A) when the mA is increased and the peak voltage and exposure time are constant, the intensity of the X-rays increases but the energy distribution stays the same; (B) when peak voltage is increased and the mA and exposure time are constant, the intensity, peak and mean energy of the X-rays increase

Quality (HVL/effective energy)
Measure of the penetrating power of the X-ray beam
Proportional to kV
Increases with constant potential
Increases with increasing filtration

Absorbed dose
Energy deposited per unit mass (Gy or J/kg)
This is equivalent to Kerma (kinetic energy released per unit mass)
Measured by an ionization chamber (effective Z of air is equivalent to soft tissue)
Alternative methods of measuring absorbed dose include:
1. dose area product meter
2. film badges
3. thermoluminescent devices (TLDs)

2.4 X-ray Interactions

Interaction with matter can result in transmission, absorption or scatter

Half-value thickness layer (HVL)

The thickness of a substance required to reduce the intensity of the beam by 50%

Linear attenuation coefficient (μ)

The fraction of the incident photons lost when travelling a unit distance (i.e. per cm)

$$\mu = \frac{0.693}{HVL}$$

Beam hardening

The X-ray beam is both wide and polyenergetic

Preferential attenuation of lower energy photons compared with those of higher energy results in the second HVL being greater than the first (increasing HVL with filtration)

Beam quality is specified by HVL in thickness of mm of Al (for example 0.3 mm in mammography compared with 3 mm in conventional units)

Mass attenuation coefficient (MAC)

A function of the mass of material traversed by the beam

$$MAC = \frac{linear\ attenuation}{density}$$

Independent of physical state but dependent on Z, E and electrons/g

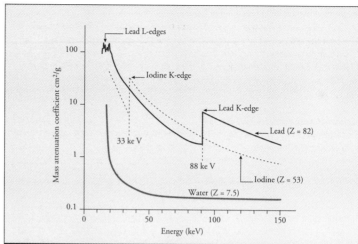

Figure 2.41 Mass attenuation coefficient as a function of photon energy; notice the sharp increase at the K-edge of lead and iodine due to the photoelectric effect at the K-edge of these materials

Attenuation

X-ray photons interact with matter, resulting in scattering or absorption
This increases with increased Z, increased density and increased thickness
There are four forms of attenuation, of which only photoelectric (PE) absorption
and Compton scattering are important in diagnostic radiology

Elastic (coherent) scattering

Interaction with a bound electron in which there is no loss of energy or ionization
Occurs for < 5% of all interactions in the diagnostic range

Compton (modified/inelastic) scattering

Responsible for nearly all the scatter produced in diagnostic radiology
Interaction between the X-ray photons and free electrons
Angle of scatter is reduced with increasing photon energy
Proportional to 1/E, density of the absorber
Independent of Z

PE absorption

Occurs if the photon energy is greater than the binding energy of the electron

The photon disappears and a photoelectron is produced; this results in the characteristic 'K edge'

Characteristic radiation is produced by the inner shell vacancy being filled by an outer shell electron

No scatter is produced

All the photon energy is absorbed; this results in an increase in patient dose

Tissue contrast is improved

PE absorption is important at low energy levels (mammography) and with elements of high atomic numbers (contrast agents)

$$PE\ effect \propto \frac{Z^3}{E^3} \times \rho$$

$$Z = \text{atomic number}$$
$$E = \text{photo energy}$$
$$\rho = \text{density}$$

Pair production

Occurs when photon energy is >1.02 MeV

Caused by interactions with the atomic nucleus and is not of importance in diagnostic radiology

Relative interaction values with atomic number and energy

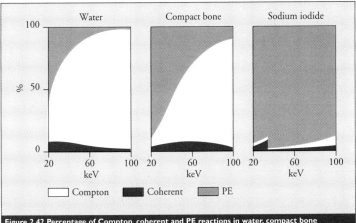

Figure 2.42 Percentage of Compton, coherent and PE reactions in water, compact bone and sodium iodide

2.5 Filters, Grids and Beam Restrictors

Filters

Reduce the patient dose (predominantly the skin dose) by approximately 80% by the absorption of low-energy photons

Two types of filtration

Inherent filtration

Tube housing (0.5-1.0 mm aluminium equivalent)

Reduces the mean beam energy, therefore reducing contrast

For mammography, an unfiltered beam (using a molybdenum filter) is required to maximize contrast, therefore a beryllium window (Z=4) is used

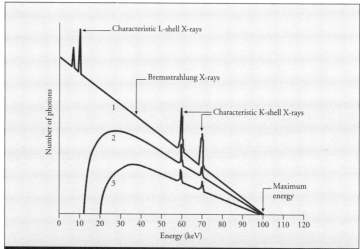

Figure 2.51 X-ray emission spectra from a tungsten target produced at 100 kV; curve (1) is the theoretical spectrum without any filtration; curve (2) is the typical spectrum with the inherent filtration of the X-ray tube and added filtration; curve (3) shows the effect of added filtration

Added filtration

Metal sheets placed in the path of the X-ray beam near the tube housing

Types of metal sheets used are aluminium (Z=13) and copper (Z=29; high-energy filtration)

A compound filter is constructed of copper with aluminium

The copper is on the tube side, the aluminium on the patient side

The aluminium absorbs the characteristic radiation of the copper filter

Disadvantage of filtration
Reduction of beam intensity
Overall reduction in contrast

K-edge (heavy-metal) filters
These remove high-energy photons, thus increasing PE and
reducing Compton interactions
Improve overall contrast but increase tube loading

Examples
Gadolinium filter — used in extremities, paediatrics
Molybdenum filter — (0.03 mm thickness) special application in mammography and
used for increasing contrast

International Committee on Radiation Protection (ICRP)
filtration recommendations
<70 kVp   1.5 mm aluminium
70-100 kVp   2 mm aluminium
>100 kVp   2.5 mm aluminium

Grids
Constructed of lead foil (0.05 mm thickness) separated by transparent spaces
Absorb scatter and increase radiographic image contrast
However, increase patient dose

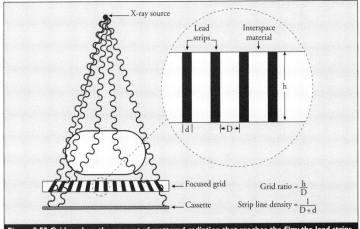

Figure 2.52 Grids reduce the amount of scattered radiation that reaches the film; the lead strips of a focused grid are designed to be parallel to the incoming beam

Grid ratio

This is the ratio of the height of the lead strips to the distance between them

Types of grid

1. linear
2. crossed (cannot be used with oblique techniques)

All grids have a focal range

Grid performance

This is based on:

1. Primary transmission (60-70%)
2. Bucky factor (total radiation absorbed by the grid; varies between 3 and 7)
3. Contrast improvement factor (increases with increasing grid ratio)

Grid cut-off

Loss of primary radiation observed with increasing grid ratio

Most commonly lateral decentering characterized by a uniform lightening of the film

If a focused grid is placed upside down, cut-off results in no exposure at the periphery

Grid selection

Compromise between film contrast and patient exposure

Examples

High grid ratio (12:1) – high kV (>90)

General purpose grids (8:1) – kV <90

Alternative to grids

Air gap

Increasing film focus distance (when using air gap)

X-ray beam restrictors

Constructed of lead
Attached to the opening in the X-ray tube housing
Control the size and shape of the beam
Reduce patient dose by decreasing field size
Reduce scatter radiation by reducing field size and increasing the film quality
Types:

    1. aperture diaphragm
    2. cones and cylinders
    3. collimators

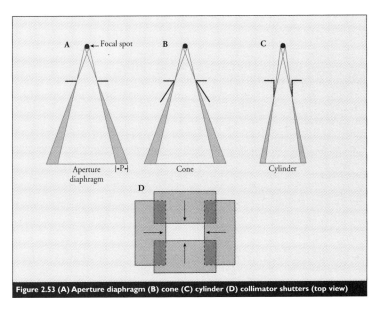

Figure 2.53 (A) Aperture diaphragm (B) cone (C) cylinder (D) collimator shutters (top view)

Aperture diaphragms produce a large penumbra (P)
Reduced by moving the diaphragm away from the X-ray target
Cones and cylinders provide accurate, fixed control of the beam
Collimators provide infinite variety combined with accurate beam control
(within 2%)

2.6 X-ray Film and Luminescent Screens

X-ray film
Film base
Invisible, flexible and provides support for the emulsion
Polyester base (150 μm)

Emulsion
Gelatin and silver halide
Gelatin maintains dispersal of the silver halide grains and prevents clumping
Silver halide consists of 90% silver bromide plus 10% silver iodide (increases the sensitivity)
Must not be a perfect crystal as photographic sensitivity would be compromised
Chemical sensitization is achieved by the addition of allylthiourea

Latent image formation
Following exposure, electrons are trapped within the sensitivity specks
This promotes the accumulation of silver ions, so forming silver atoms, resulting in the formation of a stable latent image

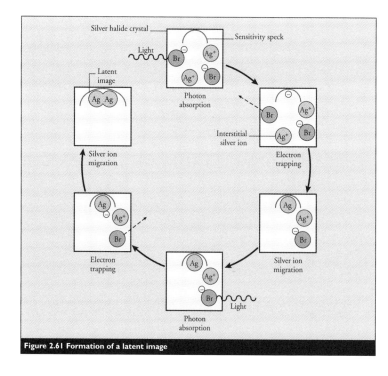

Figure 2.61 Formation of a latent image

Film processing

Development
The process converts the latent image into metallic silver specks
Image amplification $\times 10^8$
The reducing agent used is hydroquinone (pH 10) with phenidone
Timing of this stage is critical (eventually all the silver will be reduced)

Fixation
Removal of the unexposed silver halide (which reduces both image quality and stops
the permanence of the radiograph)
The reducing agent used is ammonium thiosulphate (pH 4)
Incomplete fixation produces a film with a milky appearance

Washing and drying
If this step is incomplete and the agents are not removed, the film will gradually
appear brown

Factors affecting film processing
An increase in temperature/time results in:
    1. an increase in the average film gradient (increased contrast)
    2. increased speed
    3. increased fog

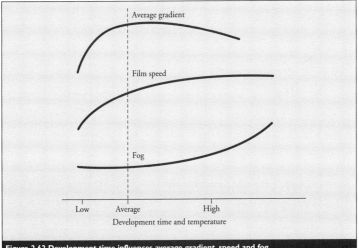

Figure 2.62 Development time influences average gradient, speed and fog

Characteristics of X-ray film

Exposure parameters

Factors influencing the quality of radiographic image, e.g. density, contrast and sharpness

These are, to some extent, under the control of the person directing the examination

Photographic density

Measurement of the film blackness

The image is produced due to variable attenuation of the X-ray beam as it passes through the patient

$$\text{Film density} = \log \left[\frac{\text{Light incident on the film}}{\text{Light transmitted by the film}} \right] = \text{Log } \frac{I_o}{I_t}$$

The diagnostic range is 0.25-2 (i.e. 60-1% transmission)

An unexposed film has a density of 0.12 = base density (0.07) + fog (0.05)

Two-sided film has a total density of the sum of the density of each emulsion

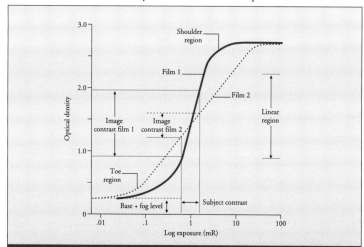

Figure 2.63 Characteristic curve showing relation between exposure and optical density for two different films; film 2 has a wider exposure latitude

$$\text{Film } \gamma = \frac{D_2 - D_1}{\text{Log } E_2 - E_1}$$

$$D = \text{optical density}$$
$$\text{Log } E = \text{log of relative exposure}$$

Defined as the maximum slope of the characteristic curve (2.0-3.5)

If γ is >1 there will be an increase in subject contrast

An increase in grain size is associated with increased speed and a small increase in γ

A small range in grain size increases film γ, whereas a large range reduces film γ

Radiographic density

Controlled by mA × sec × focus film distance (FFD)

If incorrect this will result in under-/overexposure

Radiographic (image) contrast = film contrast × subject contrast

---

Radiographic contrast is the density difference between two defined areas in a radiographic image

Film contrast

A function of the film screen combination

Affected by the characteristic curve, film density and processing, as well as by the absence or presence of screens

Subject contrast

Formed as a result of the range of the radiation intensities transmitted by the subject

Altered by kVp, density, thickness, Z, scatter and the presence of a contrast agent

Film parameters

Film speed

Reciprocal of exposure required to produce a density of 1

Film latitude

No units

Range of the log relative exposure producing an optical density range of 0.25-2.0

Increasing contrast — narrow latitude

Decreasing contrast — wide latitude

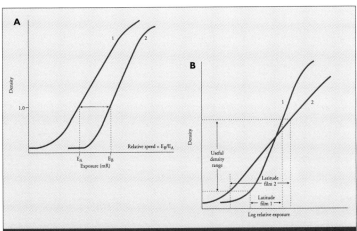

Figure 2.64 (A) The characteristic curves of two films; film 1 is 'faster' than film 2, i.e. film 1 needs a smaller exposure for the same density; **(B)** Exposure latitudes for two medical **X-ray** films; film 2 has a lower contrast than film 1 but has a wider latitude

Image quality

The accuracy of representation of each point on the object translated as a point onto the film
Affected by radiographic mottle, sharpness and resolution

Radiographic mottle

Equivalent to noise
Can be subdivided into:
1. film graininess (negligible contribution)
2. screen mottle — structural mottle (defects in the intensifying screen)
3. quantum mottle — the non-uniform pattern of light on the screen caused by photon fluctuation; this is the only noise of quantitative significance in diagnostic radiology

Sharpness

Ability of the X-ray film/film-screen system to produce a defined edge
Motion, absorption, geometry and parallax affect sharpness

Resolution

Ability to differentiate between small objects that are very close together:
1. contrast resolution is the ability to distinguish adjacent areas of different radio density (e.g. the human eye can only differentiate 11 shades of gray)
2. spatial resolution is a measure of the ability to separate images of objects placed close together

Resolution is a function of the line spread function and modulation transfer factor — both of which are measured in line pairs (lp) per mm

Examples:
X-ray films record 100 lp/mm
Screens record 10 lp/mm
Image intensifiers record 2-4 lp/mm

Fog and scatter

Both reduce radiographic contrast

Fog

Result of developed silver halide grains that have not been exposed
Increased fog with:
1. increase in film age and incorrect storage (high temperature, high humidity)
2. contaminated/exhausted developing solution
3. increased developing time/temperature
4. high film speed

Scatter

Occurs as a result of Compton interactions
Increased with increasing subject thickness, field size and kV
Reduced by collimation, grids, air gaps or compression

Luminescent (intensifying) screens

Advantages
Patient-dose reduction
Shortens exposure times, so reducing motion artefact
Improves image contrast

Disadvantage
Reduction in spatial resolution

Construction of an intensifying screen
Base
Reflecting coat
Phosphor layer
Protective layer

Phosphor layer was originally calcium tungstate
Superseded by rare-earth metals (gadolinium, lanthanum) — readily available metals with high atomic numbers

Intrinsic conversion efficiency
The efficiency of the conversion of X-rays to light by the screens,
e.g. calcium tungstate 5%, rare-earth screens (RES) 20%

Intensification factor

$$\text{Intensification factor} = \frac{\text{Exposure required without the screen}}{\text{Exposure required with the screen}}$$

The higher the intensification factor, the faster the screen
Screen speed can be increased by increasing:
1. thickness of the phosphor layer
2. crystal size
3. conversion efficiency (calcium tungstate 5%, RES 20%)
4. absorption efficiency (calcium tungstate 20-40%, RES 60%)

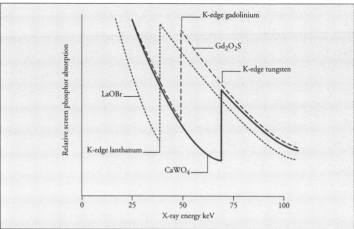

Figure 2.65 Comparison of the approximate X-ray absorption curves of CaWO₄, LaOBr and Gd₂O₂S

Emission spectra

Important to match the light output of the screen with the film sensitivity

In a calcium tungstate screen, the output is in the blue region, with a maximum of 430 nm — output corresponds to the sensitivity of monochromatic film

RES output is in the green region, with a maximum of 540 nm — corresponds to orthochromatic film

2.7 Quality Assessment

Dosemeter (Wisconsin Pentrameter)
Made of two solid-state detectors
Measures kVp and time

Ionization chamber
Can measure output, exposure and air Kerma
Can be used to check kV, mA and time exposed

Equipment assessment
Regular checks on a basic radiographic unit
Focus, field uniformity, half-value layer/beam filtration, field alignment, perpendicularity, leakage and scatter

Fluoroscopy
Routine checks are those as above for a basic radiographic unit
Additional checks:
1. input dose rate (ionization chamber)
2. image quality tests:
    gray scale — Leeds test object GS2
    low-contrast detectability — Leeds test object N3
    minimal visible detail — Leeds test object 10
    resolution — lp/mm
3. uniformity of focus (wire mesh) — Leeds test object M1

Mammography
Routine tests as applied to a basic radiographic unit
Additional tests:
1. processing — speed, contrast, base fog level
2. image quality via a phantom
3. breast dose

Computer tomography
Regular assessment of:
1. beam alignment
2. slice thickness
3. image noise
4. image uniformity (water phantom)
5. contrast and resolution (specialized Leeds test objects)
6. dosimetry (pencil ionization chamber)

Modulator transfer function (MTF)
A curve that describes the resolution capability of an imaging system
Each step of the imaging system can contribute to loss of contrast

$$MTF = \frac{\text{information in image}}{\text{information in object}} = \frac{\text{output contrast}}{\text{input contrast}}$$

Calculated using:
1. resolution test grid
2. line spread function

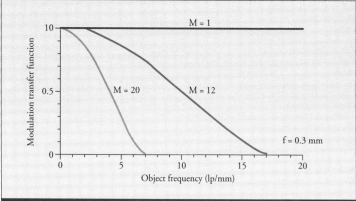

Figure 2.71 Calculated MTF curves for a 0.3 mm focal spot (f) at increasing magnification (M)

MTF allows:
1. comparison of different systems
2. assessment
3. reproducibility
4. deterioration within a system

Measurement of focal spot

Pinhole — uses magnification

Star test

2.8 Radiation Protection

Radiation effects

Stochastic (genetic and somatic)

Chance effects with no threshold, but the probability of the effect occurring is dose dependent

Examples

Cancer induction — the risk of fatal cancer is 1 in 10^5/mSv
Genetic effects — maximum risk to the foetus is during organogenesis (8-15 weeks of confinement), permanent sterility 3-8 Sv

Deterministic effects (non-stochastic)

Effects are not seen unless a threshold dose is exceeded
Severity of the effect is proportional to the dose

Examples

Skin erythema, sterilization, cataract and myxoedema

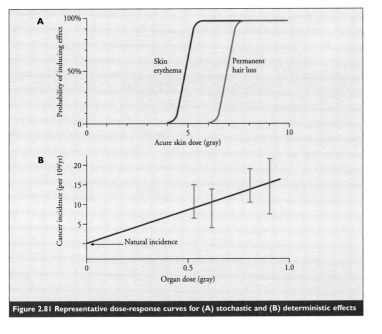

Figure 2.81 Representative dose-response curves for (A) stochastic and (B) deterministic effects

LD_{50} = the lethal dose that results in a 50% mortality = 3-6 Gy

Legislative requirements

The Ionizing Radiation Regulations, 1985
General radiation protection with maximal limit of radiation for both radiation workers and members of the public

These encompass three general principles:
1. justification
2. dose limits
3. ALARA (all exposures as low as reasonably achievable)

The Ionizing Radiation Regulations, 1988
The training of those persons physically or clinically directing a medical exposure

Medicines Administration of Radioactive Substances (MARS) Regulations
To ensure the person administrating radioisotopes to a patient has a licence to carry out the technique

The Radioactive Substance Act, 1993
To control the holding and disposal of radioactive material within the environment

The Radioactive Material Regulations, 1996
To ensure the safe transport and packaging of radioactive materials

Annual dose limits mSv

	Employees >18 years	Employees <18 years	Public
Whole body	50	15	5
Organ	500	150	50
Eye	150	45	15

Table 2.81 Annual dose limits

Females of reproductive years should not exceed 13 mSv in any consecutive 3-month period
Pregnant females should not exceed 10 mSv over the duration of a single confinement
The average staff dose within a radiology department is 1-2 mSv

Radiation units

Exposure
Measured in coulombs/kg
The amount of ionization produced in a given mass of air by a quantity of radiation

Absorbed dose
Measured in Gy
The amount of energy imparted per unit mass to a medium by the incident radiation

Equivalent dose
Measured in Sv
The product of the absorbed dose and a radiation weighting factor (Wr)
A measure of the overall biological effectiveness of a specific radiation dose
The Wr for X-rays, γ-rays and β-radiation = 1 and for particles = 20

$$Sv = Gy \times Wr$$

Effective dose
Measured in Sv
The sum of the doses in different specified organs multiplied by a weighting factor (Wt) for each organ
The weighting factors are calculated according to the ICRP 60 recommendations

Gonads	0.20
Red bone marrow	0.12
Colon	0.12
Lung	0.12
Stomach	0.12
Bladder	0.05
Breast	0.05
Liver	0.05
Oesophagus	0.05
Thyroid	0.05
Skin	0.01
Bone surfaces	0.01
Remainder	0.05
TOTAL	**1.00**

Table 2.82 ICRP 60 weighting factors

The average effective dose in the UK is 2.5 mSv:
1. 87% natural
2. 13% artificial — 11% medical

Mean effective dose due to medical diagnostic examinations:
1. the public = 1 mSv
2. hospital workers = 2.3 mSv

Procedure	Effective dose (mSv)
Chest X-ray	0.05
Lumbar spine	2.2
IVU	4.4
Bone scan	5.0
Brain scan	5.0
CT (average)	6.6
Barium enema	7.7
Heart scan (thallium)	25.0

Table 2.83 Examples of effective doses for different procedures

Areas of work

Controlled areas

An area in which an annual dose exceeding three-tenths of any annual dose limit might be received

Access is restricted; this applies to all X-ray rooms and the area surrounding a mobile unit

Supervised areas

An area in which an annual dose exceeding one-tenth but less than three-tenths of the annual dose limit might be received

Entry to the area is supervised

Systems of work

Written procedures controlling staff and public entry to controlled and supervised areas within the department

Classified worker

A worker whose annual dose may exceed three-tenths of any annual dose limit

Requires dose monitoring and regular medical checks

NHS personnel are not normally classified

Protective clothing

Body aprons with lead equivalents of 0.25-0.35 mm

Gloves with minimum lead equivalents of 0.25 mm

Dosimetry

Personal dosimetry

Legal responsibility of health authorities to protect staff from harmful effects of ionizing radiation
Required to ensure doses are kept as low as practicable and safety mechanisms work

Methods

1. film badges
2. TLDs
3. electronic personal dosemeters

Film badges

Most common method
Double-coated emulsion (one fast, one slow)
Plastic carrier incorporates plastic and metal filters
Calibrated by exposure to γ-rays (^{137}Cs at 662 keV)
Processed under controlled conditions

TLDs

Versatile personal dosemeter, especially in extremity monitoring (fingers and eyes)
Lithium fluoride in a plastic holder
Exposure results in electron trapping
Processing takes place in a light tight chamber at 400°C

Electronic personal dosemeters

A recent advancement
Very expensive and reserved for high-dose areas
Solid-state detectors or Geiger counters
Produce an immediate dose rate

Film badges	TLDs
Cheap	Expensive initial cost
Identifies type of radiation and energy of exposures	Energy independent
Permanent record	Reused
Bulky	Compact
Indirect reading	Direct reading
Range: 0.2-1000 mSv	Range: 0.1-4000 mSv

Table 2.84 A comparison of film badges and TLDs

Patient dosimetry

Two recommended methods:

1. TLDs
2. dose area product meters

Section Three
Modality-Based Physics

3.1 Specialized X-ray Imaging

Linear tomography

Simultaneous and opposite movement of anode and film about a fulcrum
Various synchronized patterns including elliptical, circular and hypocycloidal
Fulcrum determines the level of the tomographic slice

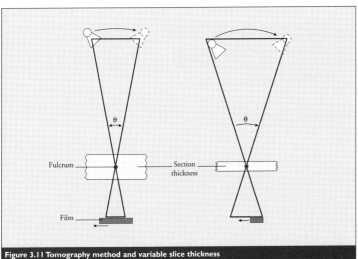

Figure 3.11 Tomography method and variable slice thickness

Slice thickness is decreased by:
1. increasing the angle of swing
2. approximating the fulcrum to the anode
3. decreasing the film focus distance (FFD)
Dose is greater than with a conventional radiograph as the time of exposure is longer

Linear tomography	Zonography
Used in areas of high inherent contrast (petrous bones)	Used to show full thickness of an organ
Large pivot angle (usually 40°)	Small pivot angle (usually 5°-10°)
Thinner slice	Thicker slice

Table 3.11 Features of linear tomography and zonography

Test tools

Angle of swing — film cassette at an angle to beam with the pivot point centred on film

Lead sheet with hole on table-top — fulcrum above sheet

Mammography

Tube design

Molybdenum target with a focal spot of 0.3 mm

Characteristic radiation produced is 17.9 and 19.5 keV

Most of the continuous spectrum is removed by the molybdenum filter (0.03 mm)

A tungsten target is used for larger breasts

A beryllium window has minimal inherent filtration and therefore transmits all the radiation produced by the tube

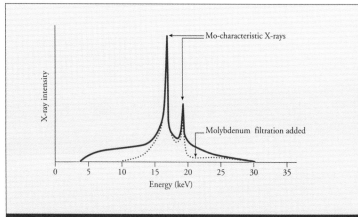

Figure 3.12 X-ray spectra from a molybdenum target at 30 kVp showing the effect of adding a molybdenum filter

Increased air gap

1.5-2 times

Grid

Always moving

Results in increased dose (x3)

Resolution

0.1 mm (5 lp/mm)

Compression
Always used unless it is not tolerated or there is an open skin wound

Advantages
Uniform tissue thickness
Decreased movement and sharpness
Decreased scatter
Decreased average dose
Decreased object film distance

Projections
Medial/lateral oblique
Craniocaudal
Lateral
Extended craniocaudal (includes axillary tail)
Paddle (magnified, valley)
Stereotactic views

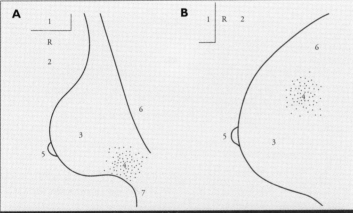

Figure 3.13 (A) Oblique view (B) Craniocaudal view
(1) Identification and date
(2) Anatomical letter in axillary region
(3) Whole breast imaged
(4) Skin pores demonstrating adequate compression
(5) Nipple in profile
(6) Pectoral muscle level with nipple and at correct angle
(7) Inframammary fold

Radiation risk
Single de novo case of breast cancer/1,000,000 women screened
Dose — 1-3 mGy
Effective dose — 0.5-1 mSv

Processing
Temperature — 36°C
Time — 3 min
Optical density — 1.7

Fluoroscopy

X-rays are converted into a light image using an image intensifier
The fluoroscopic image can be viewed directly, photographed or recorded
Components of the image intensifier:
  1. evacuated glass tube
  2. input phosphor
  3. photocathode
  4. focusing electrodes
  5. output phosphor
  6. range of size, 23-57 cm — size can be adjusted electronically

Input phosphor
0.3 mm thick
Typically consists of caesium iodide
Absorbs X-ray photons and emits light photons
Caesium iodide is used because:
  1. the vertically orientated crystals allow improved packing
  2. the thinner layer of crystals improves resolution
  3. favourable K absorption edge
     (caesium K-edge = 36 keV; iodine K-edge = 33 keV)
  4. decreased light spread, so improving sharpness resolution

Photocathode
Light photons absorbed and photoelectrons emitted
Caesium/antimony compound
Photoelectrons are accelerated across the tube by the anode potential (25-35 keV)

Focusing electrodes
Preserve the image by focusing, minifying and inverting the image
Form an electron 'lens'

Output phosphor
Formed of zinc cadmium sulphide (silver activated)
Lining of aluminium (cathode side) to prevent back scatter of light and reactivation
of the photocathode
Screen (± 10% of input phosphor)
Converts photoelectrons to light
The image from the output phosphor can be viewed:
    1. directly from a series of lenses
    2. on a closed-circuit television

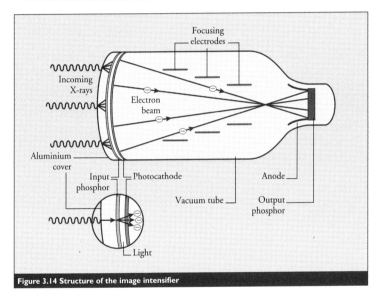

Figure 3.14 Structure of the image intensifier

Brightness gain (intensification factor)

$$\text{Brightness gain} = \frac{\text{Brightness of the output phosphor}}{\text{Brightness of the input phosphor}}$$
$$= \text{Minification gain} \times \text{flux gain}$$

Total brightness gain is approximately 5000

Minification gain

$$\text{Minification gain} = \left[\frac{\text{Diameter input screen}}{\text{Diameter output screen}} \right]^2$$

Increased gain by a factor of approximately 100

Flux gain
The increased energy of electrons attained by the accelerating voltage from the cathode to the anode
Increased gain by a factor of 50

Conversion factor
Brightness gain is not reproducible
Conversion factor is a reproducible method of measuring the gain or light output of the image intensifier

$$\text{Conversion factor} = \frac{\text{Luminance of the output phosphor}}{\text{Input exposure rate}}$$

Multiple field image intensifiers
The larger the field size, the lower the potential difference across the intensifier
The smaller the field size, the less minification of the image, so improving the resolution

Conversion of the output phosphor image
The video system comprises:
1. glass envelope
2. single plate of graphite
3. target (Vidicon/Plumbicon)
4. anode
5. cathode
6. control grid/sweep generator

Vidicon camera	Plumbicon camera
Reduces contrast by a factor of 0.8	No reduction in contrast
Improves the contrast of the fluoroscopy system	Increased resolution
Eye image lag	Decreased lag
Noise reduction	Increased noise

Table 3.12 Comparison of a Vidicon versus a Plumbicon camera

Monitor
Similar components to the camera
Vertical resolution is determined by the number of scan lines (525)
Horizontal resolution is determined by the video signal frequency (50 Hz)
Monitor brightness may be controlled by:
1. automatic brightness control — achieved by altering kV ± mA ± pulse width
2. automatic gain control — alters the sensitivity of the television monitor
A change to exposure parameters can result in increased patient exposure and increased noise

Image recording
Recording the light image of the output phosphor by photo spot and cine-radiography
Recording the television image by magnetic storage or optical disc

Image quality
Spatial resolution
Approximately 4-5 lp/mm
Affected by the blurring caused by light spread in the image intensifier
Worse at the periphery of an image
Reduced by a television system of low band width and decreased scan lines

Contrast resolution

Generally increased

Can be reduced by:

1. backward-travelling light re-exciting the photocathode (minimized by the presence of the aluminium layer)
2. incoming X-rays that penetrate the image intensifier and directly excite the output phosphor
3. ageing

Vignetting

Centre of the output image is brighter than the edges

Occurs in electron lens systems

Lag

Persistent luminescence after impinging X-ray photons have ceased

Increases with age and the Vidicon system

Digital fluoroscopy

Fluoroscopy system in which the output is digitized

Enables enhancement of the image

Reduced resolution of 'spot films' (2 lp/mm)

Digitization is achieved using an analogue-to-digital converter

Digital subtraction angiography is achieved by the acquisition of a digital 'mask image' prior to contrast injection

This can be subtracted from subsequent images following the administration of contrast solution

Enables image modification and enhancement

Provides quantitative analysis

Has improved contrast resolution

Has increased noise

Is susceptible to movement artefacts

3.2 Nuclear Medicine

Image production

Scintillation produces emissions in all dimensions
Collimators are used to select the appropriate useful radiation reaching the
detector, therefore producing an image

Gamma camera
Camera components

1. Crystal

Usually a single crystal consisting of sodium iodide activated with thallium
Size — 60 cm x 6-12 mm thick
High density, high atomic number (Z=53), hygroscopic, fragile
Takes approximately 3 months to grow
Conversion is approximately 20-30 light photons/keV (10-15%)

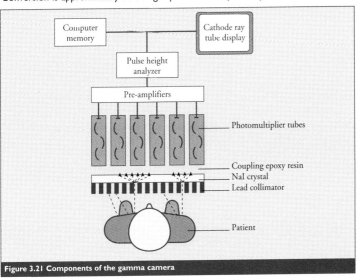

Figure 3.21 Components of the gamma camera

2. Photomultiplier tubes (PMTs)

Convert light photon energy to an electron beam
Optical couplant reduces light reflection at the crystal interface
Close packing is achieved by the hexagonal shapes
Light from the scintillation event is shared between several PMTs

3. Collimator

Improves image formation by utilizing attenuation to control the number of photons reaching the crystal

Needs to be as close to the patient as possible to optimize spatial resolution

Increases resolution but decreases sensitivity

Types: parallel, converging, diverging, pinhole

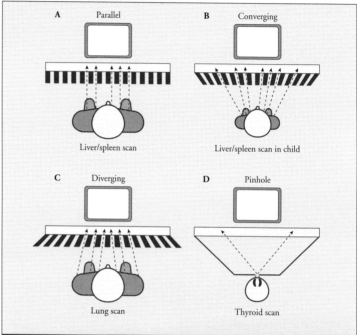

Figure 3.22 Collimators used in nuclear medicine (A) Parallel-hole collimator used for routine imaging (B) Converging-hole collimator magnifies the image (C) Diverging-hole collimator reduces image size (D) Pinhole collimator

4. Pulse-height analyser

Records the frequency distribution of the pulse amplitude

Utilizes energy acceptance windows, thus reducing scatter and blurring

Improves image quality

Increase sensitivity	Increase resolution
↑ no. of holes	↓ hole size
↑ size of holes	↑ hole length
↓ septal thickness	Small object film distance

Table 3.21 Camera sensitivity and resolution

Daily gamma-camera checks
Uniformity flood
Energy calibration
Bar phantom

Radiopharmaceuticals
Qualities of an ideal agent
Pure gamma emitter
Easily made
Localization only in the area of interest
Suitable energy range
Short half-life

^{99m}Tc (technetium)
Pure gamma emitter formed by isomeric transition from molybdenum
Available from inexpensive generators
Half-life of approximately 6 h
Energy 140 keV

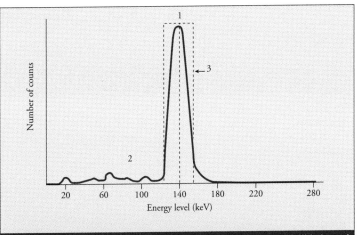

Figure 3.23 Technetium spectrum and photopeak window settings; the photopeak (1) is the result of complete absorption of ^{99m}Tc gamma rays in the crystal; Compton tail (2); the area within the dashed line (3) shows the acceptance range of a pulse height analyser set at 140 keV with a 20% window

Radionuclide production
Cyclotron: gallium[67], iodine[123], thallium[201]
Nuclear reactor: iodine[131], molybdenum[99]
Generator: [99m]Tc, 81m krypton

Half-life
Effective half-life is the sum of the physical and biological half-lives and this is always shorter than the physical half-life

$$\frac{1}{t_E} = \frac{1}{t_P} + \frac{1}{t_B}$$

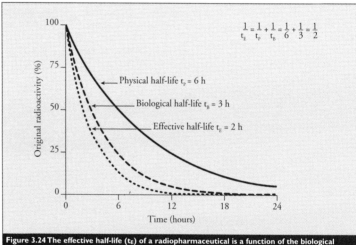

$$\frac{1}{t_E} = \frac{1}{t_P} + \frac{1}{t_B} = \frac{1}{6} + \frac{1}{3} = \frac{1}{2}$$

Physical half-life t_p = 6 h

Biological half-life t_B = 3 h

Effective half-life t_E = 2 h

Figure 3.24 The effective half-life (t_E) of a radiopharmaceutical is a function of the biological elimination (t_B) and the physical half-life (t_P)

The physical half-life is the time taken for the radionuclide to decay to half of the original value
The biological half-life is the time taken for the excretion of half of the radionuclide

Nuclear medicine techniques

Tomography

The production of sets of three-dimensional data from a series of two-dimensional projections

Achieved by the collection of a series of planar images at equal angles

Undergo filtered back projections/iterative techniques to produce coronal, sagittal and oblique views

SPECT (single photo-emission computed tomography)

Tomographic imaging used in bone scans, myocardial perfusion and cerebral blood flow imaging

Images acquired every 6° within an elliptical orbit

Improved anatomical localization and contrast resolution in comparison with planar imaging

PET (positron emission tomography)

Uses low atomic number radionuclides with very short half-lives
(e.g. ^{18}F, ^{11}C, ^{13}N, ^{15}O)

Coincidental annihilation results in the production of 2×511 keV photons at $180°$ to each other

Allows accurate localization, so improving spatial resolution (approximately 5 mm)

No collimation used

Detectors have high atomic numbers and density, e.g. bismuth germenate

3.3 Ultrasound

Longitudinal transmission of sound of >20,000 cycles/s
(one cycle/s = 1 Hz; 1 million cycles/s = 1 MHz)
It is not electromagnetic radiation, therefore it will not travel through a vacuum
Range of frequencies for diagnostic ultrasound is 1-20 MHz

$$V = \lambda \times f$$

V = velocity of sound in the conducting medium (m/s)
λ = wavelength (cm)
f = frequency (cycles/s)

The velocity of sound in a given medium is constant
The average velocity of sound is 1540 m/s through soft tissue and 4080 m/s
through bone
Velocity varies due to the difference in compressibility and density of the medium

Piezoelectric (PZ) effect

Application of an electric current causes PZ materials to rearrange their dipoles
and as a result change their shape, so producing sound waves
Heating above the Curie temperature (350°C) results in loss of the PZ effect

Types of PZ materials
Natural, e.g. quartz
Man-made, e.g. PZT (lead zirconate titanate) can act as both transmitter and receiver

Transducer

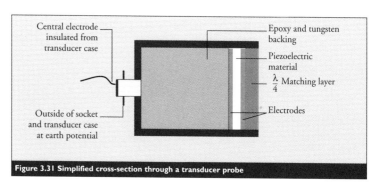

Central electrode insulated from transducer case
Outside of socket and transducer case at earth potential
Epoxy and tungsten backing
Piezoelectric material
$\frac{\lambda}{4}$ Matching layer
Electrodes

Figure 3.31 Simplified cross-section through a transducer probe

Backing layer
Formed of epoxy resin and tungsten
Absorbs sound waves that are transmitted to this layer, thus improving damping

Matching layer
Made of epoxy resin with or without aluminium powder
Axial dimension equals one-quarter of a wavelength ($\lambda/4$)
Improves the acoustic impedance mismatch, so allowing increasing energy transmission

Resonant frequency
Natural frequency of the crystal at which maximal vibration is obtained
Occurs when the wavelength of the sound produced is twice the width of the crystal
Determined by the crystal thickness
The crystal thickness is selected such that it is equal to half of the desired wavelength ($\lambda/2$)

Intensity of ultrasound
A measure of the loudness
Unit of measurement $= Wcm^{-2}$

Pulse length
Determines the axial resolution of the transducer
Dependent upon the probe frequency
Increasing frequency produces shorter pulse length, thus improving axial resolution

Quality factor (Q factor)
Measure of the purity of the ultrasound wave and the time taken to dampen the crystal (ring-down time)
A Doppler probe has a high Q factor, narrow band width, pure sound and a long ring-down time
A general probe has a low Q factor, wide band width and short ring-down time

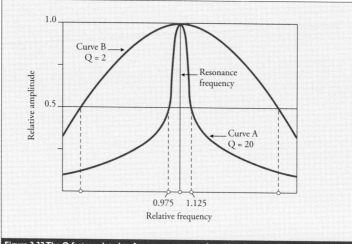

Figure 3.32 The Q factor related to frequency response for a high Q (curve A) and a low Q (curve B) transducer

Near and far fields
Fresnel zone (near field)

$$D = \frac{d^2}{4\lambda}$$

where D = length of Fresnel zone
d = diameter of transducer
λ = wavelength of the beam

The ultrasound beam is parallel in the Fresnel zone
Lengthened by:
1. increasing the frequency of the probe — improves the resolution, increases attenuation and reduces penetration
2. increasing the diameter of the beam — achieved by using a curvilinear probe, an acoustic lens or electronic focusing; the resulting ultrasound beam shows reduced lateral resolution

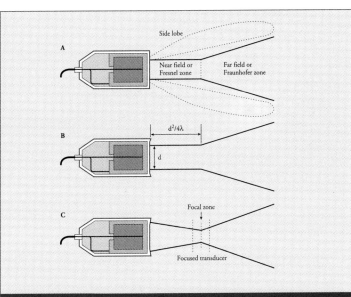

Figure 3.33 Transducer zones and focus

Fraunhofer zone (far field)
Divergent ultrasound beam
Affected by:
  1. wavelength
  2. focusing
  3. diameter of the transducer

$$\sin\theta = \frac{1.22\lambda}{d}$$
where θ = divergent angle of far zone
d = diameter of transducer
λ = **wavelength of the beam**

Acoustic impedance (Z)
The product of the density of the material and the velocity of sound within it
Unit of measurement = Rayls ($g/cm^2/s$)

Beam interactions
Reflection
Depends upon the acoustic impedance of the material and the angle of insonation
The larger the difference in acoustic impedance between tissues, the greater the
amount of ultrasound waves to be reflected
Increasing the insonation angle reduces the amount of sound waves reflected

Refraction
Refers to the change of direction of the ultrasound beam at tissue interfaces
Obeys Snell's law

Absorption
Affected by viscosity, frequency and elasticity of the medium

Transducer design
Mechanical sector
Three single elements in an oil bath
Sector image
Poor image quality
Large dead zone

Linear array
128 transducer sets firing in groups of 7
Excellent resolution
Poor depth penetration

Curvilinear
The same design as linear array but with a divergent beam
Increased depth of resolution
Decreased spatial resolution

Phased array
32/64 crystals firing simultaneously
Improved focus
Only a small footprint available (used in cardiac imaging)

Resolution
Depth (axial) resolution
Ability to differentiate between objects lying in the line of propagation of the sound wave
Only possible if the distance between the objects is greater than twice the spatial pulse length
Depth of resolution is proportional to a half-pulse length

Lateral (azimuthal) resolution
Ability to differentiate between objects lying perpendicular to the propagating sound wave
The beam must be narrower than the distance between the objects
Overcome by focusing
Lateral resolution is proportional to one-third of the diameter of the transducer

Doppler effect
Perceived change in wavelength and frequency emitted by a moving source
Movement towards the receiver results in an apparent increase in frequency whereas movement away from the receiver causes a decrease in frequency
The difference between the two frequencies is known as the Doppler shift

$$\text{Doppler shift} = \frac{2 \text{ VF } \cos\theta}{C}$$

θ = the angle of insonation
($\cos 90° = 0$, i.e. no Doppler shift at $90°$ insonation)
F = the frequency of the beam
C = the velocity of the sound in the tissue
V = the velocity at the interface

Doppler effect is increased by:
1. increasing the frequency of the beam
2. decreasing the angle of insonation

Aliasing
Ultrasound artefact occurs when the Doppler shift frequency is greater than the maximum detectable frequency
Overcome by reducing the Doppler effect, decreasing the frequency of the beam, increasing the angle of insonation or increasing the pulse repetition frequency (PRF)

Pulse repetition frequency
Number of ultrasound pulses produced per second (50-3000 pulses/s)

Nyqvist limit

$$\text{The maximum Doppler effect detectable} = \frac{\text{PRF}}{2}$$

Two modes of Doppler
Continuous wave — no depth resolution
Pulsed wave

Colour-mapped Doppler
The addition of colour flow in the mode scanning indicates the direction of flow

Duplex scanning
Coupling of Doppler and real-time ultrasound (more than 20 frames/s)

Ultrasound artefacts
Speckle
Reverberations
Mirror image
Acoustic shadowing
Acoustic enhancement
Aliasing

Ultrasound safety
Can cause damage to cells via:
1. ISPTA (intensity spatial peak temporal average), which results in local heating; not observed if intensity is <100 mWcm^2
2. ISPTP (intensity spatial peak temporal peak) produces cavitation
Sound energy should be limited to 50 joules/cm^2

3.4 Computed Tomography

Utilizes a thinly collimated, high-energy X-ray beam to obtain multiple projections of the internal structure of an object

Projections are reconstructed using a technique called 'filtered back projection' to give an image that is made up of a matrix of numbers in Hounsfield units (HU)

These are related to the attenuation coefficients of the different tissues and are represented by a gray scale

Scanning motions

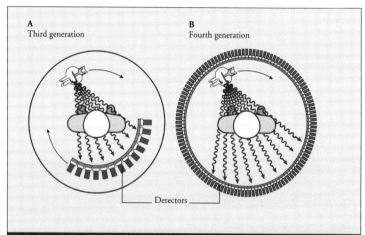

A
Third generation

B
Fourth generation

Detectors

Figure 3.41 (A) Third-generation CT scanners have a rotating tube and an array of detectors (rotate-rotate system) (B) Fourth-generation CT scanners have a rotating tube and a fixed ring of detectors (rotate-fixed system)

First generation — pencil beam, translate/rotate, one detector
Second generation — translate/rotate, multiple detectors
Third generation — rotate/rotate, gas/solid-state detectors
Fourth generation — rotate/fixed, solid-state detectors
Typical scanner values:
    120 kV
    30 mA
Focal spot of 0.6 mm

Collimators
At the tube
At the detectors:
    1. control the scatter radiation
    2. regulate the thickness of the tomographic slice

Detectors

Scintillation crystals (solid state)

Examples: cadmium tungstate, bismuth germenate, sodium iodide

Advantage

95-100% efficient

Disadvantages

Non-linear response to change in radiation intensity

Afterglow

Risk of cross-talk

Gas ionization chambers (xenon)

Use a high-density gas pressurized to 25 atm

Advantages

No lag

Linear response with varying X-ray intensities

Stable over variable temperatures and times

Disadvantages

50-60% efficient

Require precise alignment with the beam for maximum efficiency

CT number

Measured in Hounsfield units, with a range from -1000 to +4000

$$CT \ number = \frac{K \ (\mu_p - \mu_w)}{\mu_w}$$

K = magnification constant

μ_p = pixel linear attention coefficient

μ_w = linear attenuation coefficient of water

Image reconstruction

Obtained by analytical methods — two-dimensional analysis

Filtered back projection

Iterative methods

Image presentation is on a $512 \times 512 / 1024 \times 1024$ matrix

Pixel

The individual component of a matrix

Picture element

A two-dimensional representation of an area within the patient

Voxel

Volume element

The area of the patient displayed — the depth is determined by the slice thickness

Pixel brightness
Determined by the attenuation of the voxel
Represented by a gray scale of approximately 256 shades

Image display
Achieved by using appropriate window level — the central CT number
Window width — the range of CT numbers divided equally (usually) below and
above the window level

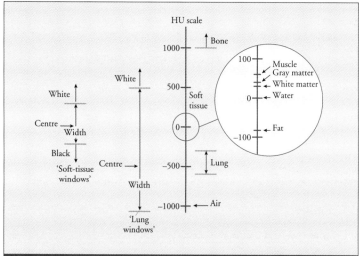

Figure 3.42 The Hounsfield Scale — windowing in computed tomography

	Window level	Window width
Supratentorial	40	80
Infratentorial	50	55
Lungs	-550	1500
Mediastinum	40	350
Liver	35	250
Abdomen	35	350
Bone	250/750	2500/3500

Table 3.41 Typical window levels and widths

Image quality

Not accurately defined for CT
Three factors are closely linked in image production:
1. noise
2. resolution
3. patient exposure

Final image represents a compromise between the best signal:noise ratio and acceptable patient dose

Noise

The limiting factor in CT performance
Refers to the variation in the number of photons detected after passing through the patient
Result of statistical fluctuations and not mathematical reconstruction
Can be reduced by increasing the number of photons (an increase in dose and increase in slice thickness)

Resolution

Function of pixel size

Spatial resolution
The ability to display two objects as separate
Improved by decreasing slice thickness and increasing matrix size (decreasing pixel size/reducing the field of view)

Contrast resolution
The ability to display areas of varying density
Improved by decreasing the noise
Compared with plain films, the spatial resolution of CT is lower but the contrast resolution is much greater

Partial-volume averaging

The CT number calculated for each pixel is a weighted average of all the constituents of the voxel
The presence of a very high attenuating material (calcium) will falsely elevate the CT number of the entire pixel

Artefacts

Patient movement — blurring in the image
Beam hardening — the average energy of the beam increases as its travels through the patient
Dense objects can produce dark bands which can be reduced by using additional filtration in the scanning gantry and by software protocols
Partial volume — see above; offset by selecting thinner slices, for example 5-mm slices in a posterior fossa
Poorly functioning detectors — results in ring artefacts in third-generation scanners that are not seen in fourth-generation scanners

Spiral scanning

Allows the acquisition of data from a large volume of the patient compared with conventional (non-helical) scanning

$$\text{Pitch} = \frac{\text{Table excursion (mm/s)} \times \text{Gantry rotation time (s)}}{\text{collimation (mm)}}$$

Advantages

Reduction in slice-to-slice misregistration
Possibility of three-dimensional reconstructions
Decreased scan time

Disadvantages

Loss of spatial resolution
Increased heat loading on the tube

	Dose (msV)
Head	3.5
Chest	9.1
Abdomen	8.8
Pelvis	9.4

Table 3.42 Average dose of CT imaging

Quality assurance

Uniformity — CT number should vary by <5 HU when measured over different areas of the scan field
Slice thickness — <10% deviation from the expected thickness
Contrast and spatial resolution measurement
Light beam alignment

3.5 Magnetic Resonance Imaging

Magnetic resonance active nucleii
Possess an odd number of protons
The size of the total magnetic moment is specific
Hydrogen atoms are used because of their great abundance and, being a solitary proton, they possess a large magnetic moment

Precession
Secondary spin caused by the external magnetic field at the precessional frequency
Expressed in the Larmor equation:

$$\omega = \gamma \beta_o$$

$$\omega = \text{precessional frequency}$$
$$\gamma \text{ (gyro-magnetic ratio)} = \text{constant of proportionality of a specific nucleus at one tesla (e.g. H} = 42.57 \text{ MHz/T)}$$
$$\beta_o = \text{external magnetic field}$$

Resonance
Occurs when a nucleus is exposed to an external field at its natural frequency
This is called the radiofrequency (RF) pulse and is delivered at 90° to the net-magnetization vector

T_1 recovery (spin-lattice relaxation)
Time constant for the recovery of 63% of the longitudinal magnetization

T_2 (spin-spin relaxation)
Time constant for the reduction in transverse magnetization to 37% of its original value

	High signal	Low signal
T_1 weighting	Fat	Air
	Methaemoglobin	Flowing blood
	Melanin	Calcium
	Proteinaceous fluid	
T_2 weighting	Water	
	CSF	
	Urine	

Table 3.51 Constant tissue signals on T_1 and T_2 imaging

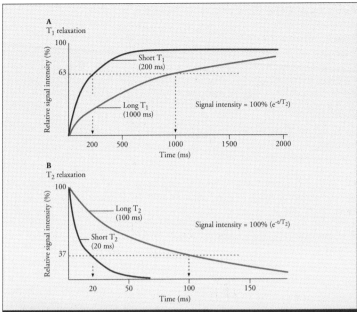

Figure 3.51 T_1 and T_2 relaxation times **(A)** The T_1 relaxation is represented as return to equilibrium of the longitudinal component of magnetization; at time T_1, the signal has grown to 63% of its maximum value **(B)** The T_2 relaxation is represented as a decrease in the transverse component of magnetization due to dephasing; at time T_2, the signal has decayed to 37% of its maximum

TR (repetition time)
Time between consecutive peak RF pulses

TE (time to echo)
Time from the RF pulse to the signal peak

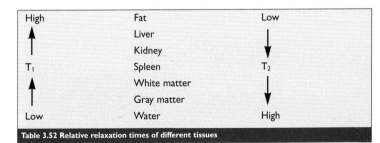

Table 3.52 Relative relaxation times of different tissues

Image weighting

$$T_1 = \quad \text{short} \quad \frac{TR}{TE} = \frac{250}{25}$$

$$T_2 = \quad \text{long} \quad \frac{TR}{TE} = \frac{2000}{60}$$

$$PD \text{ (protein density)} = \frac{\text{long TR}}{\text{short TE}} = \frac{2000}{25}$$

T_2^*

Free induction decay following cessation of the RF pulse
This is faster than T_2 decay because it comprises T_2^* decay and dephasing due to magnetic field inhomogeneities and static field produced by the patient

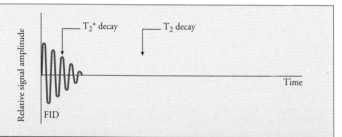

Figure 3.52 Due to magnetic field inhomogeneities, the decrease of M_{xy}, which is proportional to the relative signal amplitude, is considerably accelerated, i.e. T_2^* is smaller than T_2; FID: free induction decay

Image sequences

Spin echo
Utilization of 180° pulse to abolish the dephasing produced by magnetic field inhomogeneities

Gradient echo
Variable RF pulse according to the flip angle

Image contrast	Pulse flip angle	TE (ms)
T_1 weighted	Large (45°-90°)	Short (8-15)
T_2 weighted	Small (5°-20°)	Long (30-60)
PD weighted	Small (5°-15°)	Short (8-15)

Table 3.51 Comparison of parameter settings to achieve T_1-, T_2^*- and PD-weighted images using fast field echo imaging with relatively long TR (200-400 ms)

Advantage
Decreasing acquisition time, so reducing motion artefact

Disadvantages
T_2^* imaging, as there is no compensation for field inhomogeneities
Reduction in the signal-to-noise ratio (SNR)

Encoding
Achieved by using gradient coils so enabling:
1. slice selection
2. phase encoding — in the short axis
3. frequency encoding — in the long axis

The coil used for each coding sequence varies depending upon the plane of imaging

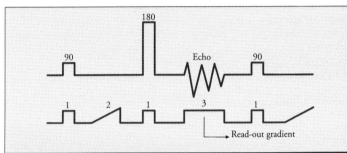

Figure 3.53 Encoding sequences: (1) slice selection (2) phase encoding (3) frequency encoding

K-space
Data information store
Does not correspond to the image

Signal-to-noise ratio
Noise is constant for both background electrical equipment and the patient
Signal output varies according to:
1. proton density
2. voxel (= field of view/matrix $\times$ slice thickness)

The SNR can be increased by:
1. increasing field of view, thickness, matrix
2. increasing TR, flip angle
3. decreasing TE

Spatial resolution
This is improved by:
1. decreasing the voxel size
2. decreasing matrix/field of view
3. thin slice selection

Fast spin echo (FSE)
Scan times are reduced by the use of an echo train
Fat remains bright on T_2 imaging

Inversion recovery (includes STIR, FLAIR)
Produces heavily T_1-weighted images

Advantages
Good SNR
Excellent T_1 contrast

Disadvantage
Long scan time

Common artefacts
Frequency-encoding axis
Chemical shift
Zipper (leak in RF shielding)
Magnetic susceptibility

Phase-encoding axis
Ghosting
Truncation
Aliasing
Magnetic susceptibility
Motion

MRI equipment
Permanent magnets
Require no power
Low running costs
Small fringe fields
Low field strengths (poor quality/long scan times)

Resistive magnets
High running costs
Fields can be switched off immediately
Large fringe fields
Low field strengths

Superconducting magnets
Expensive to buy, but cheap to run
Large fringe fields
High field strength

Shim coils
Allow correction of field inhomogeneities (approximately 10 ppm)
Require a separate power source

Surface coils
Increase SNR
Increase resolution
Decrease aliasing

MRI safety

Reported adverse effects

Mild cutaneous sensation
Involuntary muscle contractions
Cardiac arrhythmias
The sensation of 'light flashes'
Soft-tissue heating

Contraindications

Absolute

Intraocular foreign body
Pacemaker

Relative

Any metallic implants, including intracranial aneurysmal clips
Cochlear implants
Pregnancy (first trimester)
Claustrophobia

Maximum field strength

As recommended by the NRPB = 2.5 T

Fundamental Aspects of Radiology

Section Four
Pharmacology of Radiology

4.1 Contrast Media

Conventional ionic contrast media

Tri-iodinated salts of benzoic acid with variable side chains
Side chains are either sodium or meglumine salts
Sodium salts have greater side effects, including increased risk of anaphylaxis, neurotoxicity, cardiotoxicity and chemical synovitis
Meglumine salts have a larger diuretic effect and are associated with increased local vasodilatation

Low-osmolar contrast media (LOCM)

A non-ionic organic side chain is used as the cation
Half the osmolality of conventional contrast media but 2-3 times greater than that of plasma
Generally used to replace conventional contrast media
LOCM are advised in infants, the elderly, and patients with congestive cardiac failure, renal failure, diabetes mellitus and sickle cell disease
There is an equivalent rate of anaphylaxis when compared with conventional contrast media

(Note: intra-arterial injections have a 30% lower risk of reaction compared with intravenous administration)

MRI contrast agents

Alter the relaxation of protons within tissue, which also varies between tissues
Result in decreases in both T_1 and T_2 relaxation times, producing increased brightness on T_1 and increased darkness on T_2 sequences (conspicuity more apparent on T_1-weighted images)
Decrease image acquisition time

Types of MRI contrast agents

Paramagnetic
Gadolinium (Gd)
Only has a magnetic moment when a field is applied
Chelated to allow intravenous injection and is excreted via the kidneys
Gd is licensed for whole-body use and can be used in children, but not pregnancy
Can be given orally or intravenously

Supra-paramagnetic
Ferrite
Aggregation of paramagnetic ions within a crystalline lattice
Undergo rapid proton dephasing and appear black on T_2 images
Increasingly being used as gastrointestinal tract (GIT) contrast agents

GIT contrast media
Water soluble
Gastromiro (iopamidol: non-ionic), Gastrograffin (diatrizoate: ionic)

Reserved for use with suspected perforation, meconium ileus

CT imaging (2-4% solution)

Complications include pulmonary oedema (Gastrograffin), hypovolaemia, ileus and allergy

Effects are reduced by drainage at the end of the procedure

Barium sulphate
0.5-1.5 μm (Baritop): low density, low viscosity, uniform size for use in single contrast only

5-15 μm (EZHD): high density, heterogeneous size (for improved mucosal coating), used for double-contrast studies

Additional agents: antifoaming, antiflocculation and suspension agents

	w/v
Swallow examination	150%
Meal examination	250%
Follow-through examination	50%
Small-bowel enema	18%
Barium enema	125%
	(70% if single contrast)

Table 4.11 Barium dilution

Barium complications depend upon the site of utilization — perforation results in 50% mortality whereas aspiration requires only physiotherapy

Biliary contrast media

Mainly of historical interest
Derivatives of tri-iodobenzoic acid
Lipid soluble
Oral preparations have a single ring
Intravenous agents are dimers; this increases both their protein binding and toxicity
Taken up by hepatocytes
Oral agents conjugate with glucuronic acid and are excreted via the GIT
Intravenous agents remain unchanged and are excreted via the kidneys by glomerular filtration

Oral agents

Examples: Telepaque (iopanoic acid), Biloptin (sodium iopodate)

Contraindications

Hepatorenal disease, acute cholecystitis, recent intravenous cholangiogram and cholecystectomy

Complications

Pseudoalbuminaemia, abnormal liver function tests (up to 3 months), affect protein bound drugs (e.g. phenytoin)

Intravenous agents

Examples: Biligram/Biliscopan, meglumine, ioglyclamate, B, meglumine iotroxate

Contraindications

Hepatorenal disease, oral cholecystogram (within 1 week), pregnancy, Waldenström's macroglobinaemia

Complications

As for oral agents

4.2 Smooth-Muscle Relaxants

	Buscopan	Glucagon
Time of onset	Immediate	1 min
Site of action	Parasympathetic ganglia	Smooth-muscle
Dose	20 mg intravenously/ intramuscularly	0.1-1 unit intravenously
Effects (relaxes)	Lower oesophageal sphincter Pyloris Duodenum	Duodenum
Small-bowel peristalsis	Reduces	Initially reduces, then increases
Adverse effects	Anticholinergic (dry mouth, loss of accommodation, tachycardia)	Nausea
Contraindications	Glaucoma Prostatism Cardiovascular disease	Insulinoma Phaeochromocytoma

Table 4.21 Comparison of smooth-muscle relaxants

4.3 Prokinetic Agent

Metoclopramide (Maxalon)

Antagonistic to the dopamine receptors of the chemoreceptor trigger zone

Peripheral muscarinic cholinergic receptor agonist

Increases lower oesophageal sphincter tone, gastric emptying and small-bowel motility

Metabolized in the liver and excreted via the renal tract/breast milk

Adverse effects: extrapyramidal dystonia (young females) and anticholinergic effects

4.4 Local anaesthetic

Lignocaine
Prevents nerve conduction by blocking the sodium channels in axonal membranes
Maximum dose = 200 mg
20 ml of 1% solution/10 ml of 2% solution
Childhood dose = 4 mg/kg of 1% solution
Contraindications: acute porphyria, hypovolaemia, complete heart block
Adverse effects: epileptogenic and in overdose has both neurological and cardiovascular effects

Abbreviations

ACA	Anterior cerebral artery
ACL	Anterior cruciate ligament
ACoA	Anterior communicating artery
AICA	Anterior inferior cerebellar artery
Al	Aluminium
AP	Anteroposterior
ASIS	Anterior superior iliac spine
AV	Atrioventricular
CNS	Central nervous system
CP	Costophrenic
CSF	Cerebrospinal fluid
CT	Computed tomography
DJ	Duodenojejunal
FC	Fibrocartilage
FCR	Flexor carpi radialis
FCU	Flexor carpi ulnaris
FDP	Flexor digitorum profundus
FDS	Flexor digitorum superficialis
FFD	Film focus distance
FLAIR	Fluid alternation inversion recovery
FPL	Flexor pollicis longus
FSE	Fast spin echo
GIT	Gastrointestinal tract
HU	Hounsfield unit
HC	Hyaline cartilage
HSG	Hysterosalpingogram
HVL	Half-value thickness layer
ICA	Internal carotid artery
IJV	Internal jugular vein
IMA	Inferior mesenteric artery
IVC	Inferior vena cava
IVU	Intravenous urogram
LA	Left atrium
LMB	Left main bronchus
LOCM	Low-osmolar contrast media
lp	Line pairs
LPA	Left pulmonary artery
LV	Left ventricle
MAC	Mass attenuation coefficient
MRCP	Magnetic resonance cholangio-pancreatography
MRI	Magnetic resonance imaging
MTF	Modulator transfer function
NRPB	National Radiation Protection Board
OF	Occipitofrontal
OM	Occipitomental
OPG	Orthopantomogram

PCL	Posterior cruciate ligament
PE	Photoelectric
PET	Positron emission tomography
PICA	Posterior inferior cerebellar artery
PMTs	Photomultiplier tubes
PRF	Pulse repetition frequency
PZ	Piezoelectric
PZT	Lead zirconate titanate
RA	Right atrium
RES	Rare-earth screen
RF	Radiofrequency
RMB	Right main bronchus
RV	Right ventricle
SA	Sinoatrial
SMA	Superior mesenteric artery
SMV	Submentovertex
SNR	Signal-to-noise ratio
SPECT	Single photo-emission computed tomography
STIR	Short tau inversion recovery
SVC	Superior vena cava
TE	Time to echo
TFCC	Triangular fibrocartilaginous complex
TLD	Thermoluminescent device
TR	Repetition time
Wr	Radiation weighting factor

Index